The Way To Understanding Autism:

Clear, Practical Advice From A High-Function Autistic Person's Lifetime Of Experience

Copyright Information

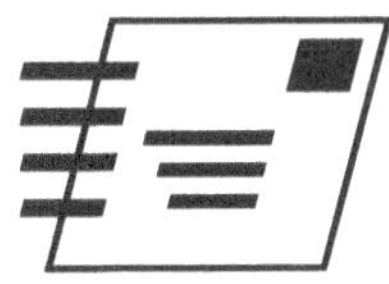

Contact Information

Wayne Blank may be contacted by email at pathfinder@keyway.ca

Make Notes!

This book is written as a "work book" of *understanding*. I urge readers to make notes throughout the text. Space is provided to do so.

I am a convinced believer in making notes because I believe that doing so enables one to not only find particular points of interest much easier later, but moreover to increase comprehension of the reading.

Contents

Preface

Welcome!

Perhaps you are someone with a beloved (but sometimes troublesome or difficult) family member for whom you wish to better understand what makes him or her think and behave as they do. You are seeking peace and happiness – for them, as well as for yourself.

Maybe you are someone who associates, by choice or by a requirement of some sort, with an autistic person as a neighbor, or at work or school, and you want to be able to get along with them better, or to become closer to them as friends.

Possibly you are a humble, open-minded medical or social professional who seeks an enlightening *inside view* of the conditions of "autism" that affect your fellow man (ironically, just like the word "man" itself, such a *singular* term as "autism" has numerous ways of making itself the constitution of many members of the multitude of humanity).

That is wonderful! Thank you for sincerely seeking more knowledge and understanding, for whatever reason, from a source that you might not have thought possible.

> ➤ **TIP** ~ Helpful points of understanding and advice such as this are included at key points in this book. Like bricks in a wall made transparent, these tips may help to reveal what most people never come to see.

I believe that this dedicated work will help you to get the clearer view that you seek because it is truly unique, perhaps somewhat *refreshingly* rare, among the now-vast market of books and videos on the subject.

This is not just a theoretical or clinical observation of other people. It is a *real life* as it has been, and is yet happening.

It is an "expertly" (i.e. a person with particular, specialized knowledge) written work because *it has been written by someone with autism* - who is nevertheless quite able to communicate his now-substantial amount of knowledge and awareness of the subject to those who wish to learn from it.

> ➤ **TIP** ~ Communicative (able and willing to communicate) autistic people tend to be "plain speakers." They simply speak, quite literally, what they truly think. An offense is rarely intended – *but is often the inadvertent result*. When reading this book, or speaking with any autistic person, please keep that inadvertent factor in mind (more about that "Mr. Spock" literal bluntness in a later chapter).

I am a healthy, independent, self-supporting person with autism. That too is an important lesson about the condition - perhaps for many, the most important revelation of all.

A friendly warning! Be ready for some *pleasant* surprises and discoveries that will make autism less of a mystery to you. In so doing, you could even come to realize some things about yourself, as I did.

Enjoy!

Why Was This Book Written Now?

I probably would not have written this book if I were much younger. There are two primary and practical reasons for that as-it-happened occurrence. It was not a simple matter of choice or curiosity on my part.

The first reason is that *I did not specifically know* about the autism, as such, until just a few years ago, after age 55. It was discovered by accident while trying to prove to someone who I cared very much about that I was not affected by something else. I was, in effect, forced into the unexpected discovery. I will detail that in a later chapter.

I always sensed that "the world" was *seemingly* somehow different, but it was only relatively recently, with that startling and in-retrospect now life-defining and self-explaining discovery, that I became aware of the reason. *I was different in the world such as it is*.

> ➤ **TIP** ~ Autistic people generally regard themselves as "living in their own world" because they think it normal and natural that everyone else does too. It is *not* a matter of the generally foreign-to-autism personality trait known as "attitude." It is simply a matter of *perception* as the view *outward* happens to be.

The finding was not exactly like Hans Christian Andersen's *The Ugly Duckling* (in the original Danish, *Den grimme ælling*) fairy tale in which a scorned and ostracised member of the barnyard flock discovered that it was not a duck at all. I can nevertheless relate to that bird - even though I was never scorned and ostracised in such a way.

I was "left alone" to *be* alone (notice how common terms can have different meanings, or multiple meanings, to each person). For me, it was *easy*.

I do know though what feeling different (a self-conscious awareness), or being made to feel different (by others), or even having been made to feel different (having been born this way) are *all* like. It was, and is, however not a bad feeling to me. I am quite happy as I am. I always have been. I don't see any reason that I would not want to continue to be *me*.

By the way, some are of the opinion that Hans Christian Andersen himself was in some way, or ways, autistic. If so, there may have been a greater message and lesson in his *The Ugly Duckling* narrative. Maybe he consciously intended it as such in its creation. Perhaps he did not. However, it is *there* in the eyes of many who *live* it.

Suddenly A New World

It was a "bolt from the blue" made-certain awareness, despite all of the signs that had been there, even to semi-conscious about it me for a lifetime, that it was not as much "the world" as it was me was a shocking and humbling experience.

To this day, I find it astonishing – although probably not such a shock or surprise to those who have known me for any length of time. For some or most family, friends and acquaintances, it must have been *obvious*, while to me, it was yet *oblivious*. It is not so anymore.

I nevertheless always knew that there was something different, to use the common term, not "normal" – a word that simply means what most people are, or have been trained or conditioned to be.

The majority-defined *democracy* of "normal" does not of course actually refer to, or guarantee, what is right or wrong in reality. It just declares what most people are - and what everyone is then expected to be.

If most people had green skin, that would be the natural, "normal" way of being human."White" or "black" or "yellow" would be abnormal – or shall we say, *not average*.

If most people have been "educated" (I won't use the words *brainwashed* or *indoctrinated* because I don't think that it is quite that simple) to venerate a particular symbol of some sort, religious or political, it would be politically "normal" to do so – and abnormal, to the point of being offensive to the others, not to be of that popularized single mind view. More about that what I call "group autism" later – and by that I *don't* mean a "group home" for autistic people!

> **TIP** ~ Autistic people are generally *normal in their own eyes*. They do not
> realize that anything is "wrong" with them – *if* indeed there actually is
> anything "wrong" with most of them at all. Their defensive reaction (that is
> often used as a justification or pretext to further regard them as having a
> problem – when the difficulty can sometimes be just as much in the
> observer and judge of the autistic person) is simply a response to those
> who violate their space in an uninvited or perceived threatening way.
> Friends are welcome. Aggressors are not welcome. *Everyone* wants his or
> her at-home-in-me space. Don't *you*?

"Neurotypicals"

I actually find the present term "neurotypicals", in referring to "normal" people who are
not autistic, a little humorous. I think that it is somewhat right, but not exactly in the way
intended. I think that it is, or will be, a backfiring term, sooner or later. *It's an invitation
for reality to strike*.

Perhaps they are setting themselves up for a surprise someday, but hopefully, a good
one that will enable them to grow and appreciate more of the diversity of the *entire*
world around them – and that it does not end at *their* horizon. I wish them the best and
hope for their happiness.

Seeing happy people makes me happy too – even more so now after I discovered that I
am autistic. It's all much more valuable and worthwhile now.

"Normal" is relative. It is simply a matter of majority versus minority in a given time and
place. Somewhere or sometime else, the normal may be abnormal. Step across a man-
made physical or psychological border and suddenly you could find yourself regarded
as foreign, alien or abnormal. Travelers do it all the time.

Minorities Of One

With the autism awareness, I very suddenly felt like a minority person in a society made
for and run by a "normal" majority – even though the majority itself is composed of
"minorities" who regard themselves, as a whole, "normal."

I used to think that I was one of those "others" (even though I continue to be part of
various other "normal" majorities) but I never actually was. Surprise, surprise.

> ➤ **TIP** ~ Autistic people are a *minority* very much like any other. In most cases, asking about and respecting what is *naturally different* about them is much more productive than merely judging what is "wrong" with them. Everyone is "human." Before judging the burdens that others have been given to carry, go and have a careful look at yourself, and your life, in a mirror. Be honest with what, not just who, you see looking back at you.

My opinion about that may be one of the somewhat comforting compensations that I have embraced to be more at peace with *what is normal to me* and all like me – and I now know that there are many such people.

Were you waiting for me to say that because you were already thinking about it? Good! It shows that "normal" and autistic people can communicate and understand each other. That result is the primary intended purpose of this book – and proof in itself that the means that I offer *works*.

I suppose that I could be more defensive about it too, and sometimes I am - *unapologetically* so (as you will probably notice if you haven't already too). Perhaps that's a leftover from my previous life (as it sometimes seems) as a "normal" person.

Overall though I prefer to explain as best that I can what it is like from my own lifetime of experiences. I may be fortunate to be able to attempt to do that, while many of the other people "on the spectrum" obviously are not. That is the paradox.

> ➤ **TIP** ~ Many of those who should explain autism best cannot explain it at all. The problem is not behavior as much as it is communication.

However, enough on that point, for now. More later.

Autism's Biography

While much of this book is about my life, the book is *not* really about me. It is not a biography as much as it is about the autism that made me, *me* – and others as they are. *Perhaps it is* somewhat of *autism's biography* played out on one person's life stage.

I offer myself, my experiences, as a learning tool for the readers to use if they wish to do so. I hope that you do because I believe that the lessons are a beacon to anyone who wishes to see a guiding light that actually lives what he's explaining. That is not making something dramatic. It is just stating something as it is in reality.

Honest critics are welcome. I have found them to be useful in seeing what I cannot, or have not yet, come to see. From that, if they are correct, good things can be done.

While reading this book, I reiterate to please keep in mind as well that a classic trait of autism is *directness*. Some may regard that as opinionated, dogmatic or even arrogant (as we will cover in a later chapter, that is how my autism was discovered – while attempting to prove a layperson's "diagnosis" incorrect – which it was), but I am merely expressing myself in the matter-of-fact, unbiased way that is natural for *me*.

No offense what so ever is intended in my "Let the chips fall where they may" manners.

Pride and Prejudice

The second reason that this book was not written much sooner is a reactionary extension of the first. Such a frank, in-places personally embarrassing ("Why in the world would you make *that* publicly known?" is a question that some might ask while reading this book) and at-times brutally honest (in a "Forest Gump" sort of way – more about some of those fictional characters with *real-life displays of autism* a little later too) exposure of one's personal self would almost certainly, in a wide range of ways, be very costly and troublesome to a younger person – employment, business, dating and the general attitude toward someone who is different in any way that isn't "normal."

I have experienced a little of it myself since I made my autism public (immediately after it was made public *to me* too) – as much as I sensed, or bothered to notice. I will not use the word "discrimination," at least not in the way that it is commonly used, because I do not think that is what it is – as much as it is merely the human, all humans, tendency to fear and run from what is not yet known or understood.

Why Do People Fear And Hate Others?

Discrimination may be a primal defense mechanism in recognizing potential danger. It can be done innocently (e.g. avoiding people of bad or criminal behavior or those who are blatantly threatening in word or stance), or it can be done maliciously (e.g. racism or political and religious persecution – more about that later in the shocking origin of the term "autism" itself).

I am not an anthropologist, but I am, like everyone else, able to discern what I like or do not like – or who I like and who I do not like. That is everyone's moral right, providing that it does not become an aggressive moral or legal *wrong* to other people.

I suppose that I did it to others as much back then (but certainly not as much now) as others do it to me now. Along with the "surprise, surprise" may have come *justice, justice*. Good!

If it balances the scale more, it is welcome. It is a growing, not merely up (which can simply mean *more* of what was done earlier i.e. "the same ole, same ole thing"), but *away* from a lesser self. A journey of genuine distance, not of merry-go-round circles.

Much more bias and prejudice might come with the publishing of this book, but so be it if that happens. I am at the point in this life when doing what I believe is genuinely important is all that matters. As people who get older come to appreciate, what cannot be lost cannot be taken *either*. Some might define that as true *freedom*.

I would much rather enlighten interested others as best I can now than to waste precious time and effort by foolishly alienating them by enraging them with deliberate hostility. Anyone can choose that low road to no where. I prefer not to do so.

Real Life Knowledge and Advice – Not Just Medical Opinion Or Dogma

I am not a medical professional of any sort. I hold no degrees in medicine, psychiatry, psychology or any of the fields of health that declare themselves to be the credentialed (i.e. authority created by members of an organization or profession to be provided to themselves for their own power and rule over others) official authors and custodians of autistic theory.

This book is not about providing medical advice about autism. It is about *understanding actual experience*, not the treating or "curing" of it by those who have never experienced it. Therein exists *their* "problem" in effectively helping those that they seek to treat. *Understanding*, not just knowing.

I can only provide advice about the condition as I have myself experienced it. Therefore, although it is written about me, it is only through and by means of that experience, from the earliest childhood memories to the present, that I believe, I comprehend the condition, now, very well indeed. This is about a *real* person, with *real* autism.

Revealing The *Why* Of The Behavior

I believe that much of what I frankly and honestly describe in these pages will be very familiar to those who live or otherwise have contact with the autistic community. I also suspect that the *why* of the behavior will be a useful basis of learning about what is actually happening.

What seems obvious may not exist at all. Dogmatic illusions - medical, political, religious or of any other kind - can seem very real, particularly to those who *want* to believe them.

I hope that this book provides a *reality* view that many people seek. I urge you to read it *all* – any particular chapter, or this Preface, are not complete without the specifics described throughout the whole work.

Height And Depth Of The "Spectrum"

I should also like to emphasize that autism, and its related conditions, are indeed a "spectrum." It is very wide and very deep in how the *same*, perhaps *single* (maybe the cause of autism is itself "autistic"), the internal source may affect people to a wide range of degrees. Perhaps the variability of the intensity of a single force that is what the "spectrum" really is.

I believe that I have a genuine understanding of the behaviour patterns and impulses that, as with all "who have the focus" (I will explain that later), makes me far more of an expert, a practical specialist, if you will, than those who merely try to treat the inside from their view of the outside. With all due respect (which I do) to them and their professions, *living it is really knowing it.*

Like the surface of an ocean, there is much that can be seen and understood about what happens at or is bubbling from the surface. But only those who have, not just seen it, but been and lived in the vast realm below the interface of where the water meets the air, can truly know what they are talking about when they explain the beauty and the ugliness, the love and the fear, the peace and the dangers, of what is on the other side of the no depth or height line at the surface.

To be fair, and as would seem obvious, perhaps those with autism (I will use that simple summary word for the "spectrum") do not really very well understand what they cannot see on the other side of them either. However, we will let the medical professionals take care of that. That is *their* side of the experience.

A last note about being defensive. If you have experienced any sort of discrimination in your life, then you understand why some with autism, after they realize that it is happening, may find it quite offensive. But that is "natural" for *everyone.*

It does not matter what the subject of the bias happens to be. The feelings of the ones (I emphasize the word *ones* there – a plurality of very singular people) being subjected to it are the same. No one likes to be looked down upon by a fellow human being. *No one.*

A "Walk A Lifetime In My Shoes" Method Of Understanding

So, as we begin the reading, be ready for some surprises along the way. *Good* ones!

"Way" literally means *road* (i.e. highway, freeway). It defines a route, a journey from a beginning point to the desired destination.

By beginning to read this book, you have chosen to a make a journey of discovery made possible by the sights along the way. As an autistic person, I offer my life's experiences, good and bad, happy and sad, as those sights that may serve as guides toward the destination – a better understanding of what is truly a complex, but not mysterious or unfathomable, condition.

I sincerely hope that this book is helpful to you and the autistic people that you care about and love, regardless of what side of the condition that you have found yourself. I know that it helps me to write it.

Wayne Blank

(Yes, "Blank" is my real name; it's German-Dutch)

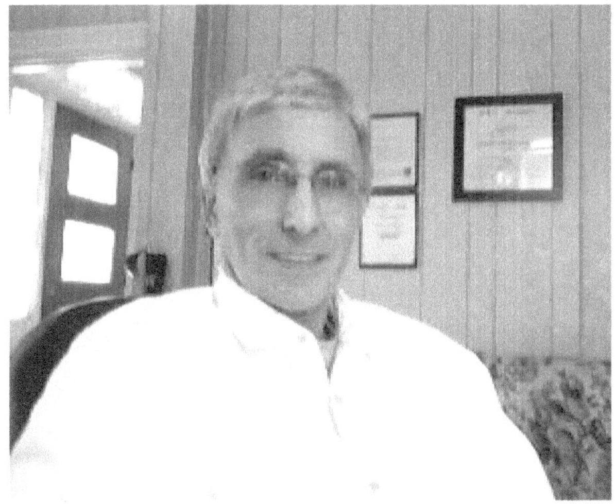

Wayne Blank

Section 1: Causes and Effects Of The "Spectrum"

Chapter 1: What Does "Autism" Mean?

The Shocking Origin Of "Autism"

What does autism supposedly mean? Where and when did the word originate?

The history might shock you. It most surely shocked me, *deeply*.

In 1910, a German-speaking psychiatrist in Switzerland, Eugen Bleuler (1857-1939), used the Greek word, pronounced *autismus* (which was translated into English as *autism*) in his opinion of one of the visible symptoms of schizophrenia. His use of the term was the basis for what is commonly known as autism today (even though autism is *not* schizophrenia).

Many find it appalling that Bleuler was also a proponent of forced sterilization of those judged by him, and others like him, to be "abnormal." It was a view that the evil fiend Adolf Hitler adopted a few years later as part of the murderous Nazi supposed "purification" of his Germanic race.

A quote from Bleuler's *Textbook of Psychiatry* (1924).

> "The more severely burdened should not propagate themselves. If we do nothing but make mental and physical cripples capable of propagating themselves, and the healthy stocks have to limit the number of their children because so much has to be done for the maintenance of others, if natural selection is generally suppressed, then unless we will get new measures our race must rapidly deteriorate."

Bleuler would apparently have "euthanized" actual autistic people too (others of his like mind actually did, as we will get to in a moment) for what he obviously regarded as a genetic-caused condition – no environmental or vaccine-damage causes of autism in Bleuler's "pure race" theories!

Bleuler's writings also included some bizarre and morbid views of human sexuality. One can only guess to what degree he was projecting himself in that regard onto his very warped view of others. I believe, based on his behavior and opinions, that the man had some very serious psychological problems.

Johann Asperger

Another very shocking chapter in the history of autism followed along in the same era. The Bleuler influence and connection continued on to one of the most famous names in the world of autism study and care.

The present-day use of the word originated in the late 1930s from Johann ("Hans") Asperger (1906-1980), a pediatrician at the Vienna University Hospital, who used *Bleuler's word* in describing children that he said were *autistic psychopaths.* The now-famous Asperger Syndrome, also known simply as Asperger's, was named after him.

As with Bleuler, Asperger had a lurid, direct connection to Adolf Hitler's Nazi regime "race purity" movement. Most people find that absolutely appalling about him, considering his now respected and revered place in the world of medical and social professions.

European historian Edith Sheffer, the author of *Asperger's Children: The Origins of Autism in Nazi Vienna* (2018), wrote that Asperger was an actual operative within Hitler's Nazi dictatorial government in which he was directly responsible for sending hundreds of children to be "euthanized" at the Am Spiegelgrund children's clinic in Vienna, Austria. That Nazi child-killing program had the official "public health" title of Aktion T4.

Adolf Hitler was himself actually a native of Austria, not Germany. Hitler spent his on the street hobo years in Vienna after his widowed mother's death from breast cancer in her mid-40s. Klara Hitler was thereafter no longer around to feed and house her then-adult dependent son.

It is unfortunate that Adolf Hitler was not treated, while he was there, for *his* severe psychological malfunctions, whatever they were. It could have saved millions of innocent, healthy people, including many with autism, who were tortured and murdered by a very sick man who declared that his victims were the sick ones.

In 2018, Herwig Czech, a historian with the Medical University of Vienna, also described Asperger's Nazi connections in an article in the journal *Molecular Autism* (published April 2018):

> "Asperger managed to accommodate himself to the Nazi regime and was rewarded for his affirmations of loyalty with career opportunities. He joined several organizations affiliated with the NSDAP (although not the Nazi party itself), publicly legitimized race hygiene policies including forced sterilizations and, on several occasions, actively cooperated with the child 'euthanasia' program."

I find that absolutely outrageous! Those now-respected men were apparently *not* honest scientists or ethical "first, do no harm" medical professionals. Like Hitler himself, they were opportunistic raw-minded racists and moral bigots. That grossly-shameful *criminal* part of their history has since been mostly whitewashed and ignored by the popularized autism movement of today.

In the years after the Second World War (1939-1945), Asperger became more publicly humane in his view of autistic people. Honest-minded *thinking* people might wonder if Asperger would have accommodated himself to his supposedly changed mind if Hitler had not lost the war and committed suicide with his few remaining cronies.

Many of Hitler's other followers thereafter also declared that they were not actually Nazis after all in a clumsy, but generally accepted, attempt to keep themselves from being prosecuted for war crimes and crimes against humanity. The "I was just following orders" excuse. Again, "the same ole, same ole."

Moreover, as you can see, the genesis of the term was to describe schizophrenics and psychopaths – very different conditions, apart from any passing, coincidental symptoms that someone may decide that they are seeing.

Time has proven the often-malignant opinions of *some* of the pioneer "experts" (to be fair, there were, no doubt, many good medical professionals too) on the subject of autism *wrong* – as much in their theories, as in *their* horrendous state of mind.

To me, what they really were, on a personal level, then on a professional level, is absolutely horrifying and disgusting.

A More Humane Definition

For those not in the medical professions, the term is usually first encountered in those that they love, rather than coldly as "subjects" at some clinic. Less dehumanization, but often just as much misunderstanding, albeit well-meaning for the most part.

For an ordinary person, the *Oxford Dictionary*, for example, now simply defines "Autism" as *"a mental condition in which a person has great difficulty in communicating with other people. Origin from the Greek autos, self"*

Although much more benign, that is obviously still an outsider's view and definition of the condition. How would an autistic person regard that definition? Reasonable? Or arbitrary and judgmental? I suggest the latter.

> ➤ **TIP** ~ According to the definition, *"a mental condition in which a person has great difficulty in communicating with other people,"* I am not autistic. *But I am.* So are millions of others – a few very well known (as we will get to), but most unknown. Beware of definitions, from any source, that offer to define *everyone*. They don't.

Personally, I could easily find it somewhat condescending, although I am not saying that the writer(s) of that later definition meant it to be so. Unlike the very disappointing toxic arrogance of Bleuler and Asperger (that transcends time – many still have their "spirit" today), they were more just products of their era and place, regardless of its to-a-degree, depending on any particular autistic person, basis of accuracy.

There is a profound difference between the "leaders" and their followers who reduce themselves to parroting dogmatic theories. But beware of whose coat tails that one rides along on!

Referring back to the Preface, regarding the reason that I wouldn't have written this book earlier (if I had known that I had the condition), it verifies that sort of prejudice, at times throughout the past century, *deadly* prejudice, that is, I believe, more often a greater handicap than the condition itself. Some may perhaps use it as an opportunity to vent their hate for *everyone*.

I find it extremely difficult to respect or look up to such "professionals" with minds and attitudes like that. I *hope* that such people were in a minority in their own time, as well as now.

Bleuler and Asperger seem to me like a proverbial dentist with a mouth full of bad teeth – behaviorally repugnant and hypocritical in what they profess.

Perhaps those with that attitude are handicapped or developmentally challenged from *their* shallow view of what they're actually observing. Something is indeed very wrong with them.

I do not mean to be harsh, judgmental or aggressive in the historical reality that I have written here. But the facts are the facts. I am only being straightforward, yes, perhaps blunt, in what I honestly believe in view of them.

That is one of the classic symptoms of autism - maybe one of the best ones for the common good. Being able to recognize evil and having what it takes to say so is *not* a bad thing.

Why Can *You* Communicate?

A reader of this book might point out however that I do not seem to be having any problem communicating with you, the *reader*, which is correct.

However, if I were to sit down and have an in-person conversation with that same reader, it might be awkward for one or both of us. I am friendly and I like people, but I am not a conversationalist. I stopped trying to be one when I came to peace with the idea that "a fish should not try to fly." It is not the way they are, except in fantasies and frauds.

"Get Back To Me"

I have always found it particularly difficult to reply to communications, not because I do not want to, but because it is perhaps more of a formal and stressful effort for me. I am not very good at "chit chat" or brief one-liners.

That known from experience pressure makes it an ordeal that further makes it even more difficult to reply. So too the knowledge that my reply will likely be "read" in a way or *tone* that was not intended makes it even more of a blockage to replying. It escalates into an impossible situation, so I simply write it off (no pun intended) with the self-consoling belief that not replying would actually do less damage than a reply would anyway.

I can, and do, reply, but it might take much longer than most people are willing to wait before they assume that they are being snubbed – *which they are not*. For me, an expected reply is a friendship destroyer.

> ➢ **TIP** ~ The autistic characteristic of not replying is not simply refusing to do so, or ignoring what is said to them. It may be just a matter of "*when* I can" or "*If I can*."

Some have never been answered, even though I really wanted to, and from that have assumed the same as the person who was instrumental in my discovering that I am autistic. More on that in a later chapter.

"Auto"

The word "auto" itself is also interesting. Most people are familiar with it from the word automobile, which means *self-moving*. However, such vehicles still need a driver or they do not move at all. Horses, which were replaced by automobiles for transportation, are not automobiles because they have a living brain.

> ➢ **TIP** ~ Autistic people, like everyone else, are "self-moving" too. It is just that their driver, often with no choice, travels along a very precise route. Any road will *not* do.

I agree that "spectrum" has been used to describe the wide, *very wide*, range of how the (I believe) single condition is experienced to a lesser or greater effect. I agree with that term in principle, but I use "autism" here because I believe that it is the basis of it all.

Life In Orbit

The only other word that I think would be more accurate than spectrum is *orbit*. Like electrons orbiting the nucleus of an atom (it is the magnetic force of the positively charged nucleus that makes the negatively charged electrons orbit, regardless of how differing in distance or velocity their orbits may be), everyone on the spectrum orbits the single focus of what makes them so. The closer in, or the farther out, is the actual spectrum. Regardless of the velocity or distance, a single force draws them inward.

It seems to me that autism is more of a three-dimensional orbit that requires a globe to illustrate, rather than a two-dimensional spectrum that can be displayed on a flat electronic surface or a piece of paper.

There are many kinds of plants, but they all have a root system that works in the same way as the very life basis of their existence. To me, that is also more like an orbit than just a spectrum. So too, autism.

This book is intended to present what "autism" means to those who are autistic. In so doing, I hope that the reader will see how and where the clinical definitions are reasonably accurate, and where, at times, *they really do not know what in the real world that they are talking about in their declarations.*

> **TIP** ~ Sometimes, toxic-minded people like Bleuler and Asperger become far more influential than they ever should have been. Fame or power is no guarantee of being *right*. Sometimes they merely enforce what is very *wrong*.

Chapter 2: The Cause Controversy

Genetics or Environment? Ancient Malady Or Modern?

There are many in the present era who are of the opinion that autism is a relatively new, or even just a modern-day affliction (i.e. something that has happened to someone, as opposed to how they already are from birth). Perhaps they have a somewhat personal motive for that opinion, conscious or subconscious.

If someone has an autistic child, it may be easier to innocently "blame" (yes, I will use that word) present-day pollutants, or the use of vaccines, rather than view the condition as having existed for centuries or millennia – so thereby those with autistic children may be the genetic couriers of it.

The latter could seem to affix responsibility more on genetics (the Bleuler and Asperger view – the reason that they wanted to sterilize or "euthanize" autistic people), or the actions of the parent.

To me, it is an irrelevant concern. I do not blame anyone. I see no valid, honest or loving reason for others to do so. What happens ("chance to be or do something, without intention or causation") has happened ("come into being; become reality").

> ➤ **TIP** ~ Regardless of its cause(s), autism is not a blamable condition. There is no guilt without bad *intent*.

If autism is genetic, would an autistic child be able to justify their at-times troublesome behavior within a family by saying "I didn't make me autistic, *you* did"? Apart from the fact that an unwilling or unknowing carrier is not a creator, it would do nothing but to cause suffering for the *innocent*.

> ➤ **TIP** ~ Autism *is not* anyone's fault.

For reasons mentioned earlier, I did not find the word "autism" in my old 1940s *The Consolidated Webster Encyclopedic Dictionary*. The reason for that is obvious - the specific term only began to be used by the Nazis and their like-minded medical professionals about that time, but it is listed in my present-day *Oxford English Dictionary*.

Does that mean that the *Oxford* is more complete and exhaustive about the *condition*? I do not think so. Some other appropriate word, or words, fitting to a particular part of the spectrum, for it *should* be there in the older dictionary. But it seems not to be.

Does that imply then that the condition was so relatively rare before a century ago that words for it were not included in a quality college-level dictionary? It could be.

Why did that *term* for it have to be invented in the first half of the twentieth century? Why so seemingly late? Why by people with the philosophy of Bleuler and Asperger, of all people? Their term "autism" began as an excuse to sterilize or even kill people!

Perhaps we will come upon the revealing answer as we proceed through this book.

Most Of Those With The Answers Can't Communicate Them

It may be that the reason that a single word for it cannot be found is that a single word for it *is not enough*. Autism is indeed experienced in a very wide range. It truly is a spectrum. That in itself might indicate that there are multiple causes of the condition, some producing a debilitating condition, while others produce a "genius."

> **TIP** ~ "Autism" notwithstanding, no single word is enough to explain or describe it. There is no "one size fits all" answer to practically any question about autism. Humans overall are individuals. Autistic people may be even *more* so.

For some, it is an impairing handicap, while for others it is, in some ways, a blessing. I could regard myself among the latter – but with a lot of trouble, for others and myself, along the way. We will get to that.

I do believe however that regardless of how it is manifested, multiple causes or not, all people with autism, regardless of their age, are experiencing very much the *same state of mind*. It is just a matter of how high the autistic "volume" is set.

The greatest paradox of it may be that those who are best qualified to communicate with others of the same condition are unable to communicate with anyone – not only because some cannot speak at all, but because such difficulty in expression is the definition of the condition itself. There are a few who are exceptions to that.

If "normal" people could communicate, without any difficulty, with the autistic they would have to be autistic themselves – and vice versa. I do believe however that there are certain keys to *the common ground areas* that will open the door sufficiently to that place, regardless of how heavy and locked it may seem.

The List Of Possible Causes Is Also A Spectrum

The cause, or causes, or complexity of variable causes of autism may be a matter of much controversy – such as when it actually develops, whether in fetal development or in the first few years of life.

The now-lengthy list of professional guesses of possible causes includes heritable genetics, a failure of the fetus to develop in a "normal" way (the same used to be said about, for example, homosexuality, before it became politically incorrect to suggest that the "gay brain" did not develop sufficiently beyond its feminine, that is *effeminate*, genesis), for whatever reason, or exposure to a wide range of toxins or infections (of mother or child – separately or together), before or shortly after birth.

I will make no attempt to dogmatically declare a cause (although I will make an educated-by-experience guess at the end of this chapter). I can only explain my own actual experience.

I *knew* (I will qualify that in a moment) of no other family member, past or present, with the condition - at least not to the level that I experience it.

My brother and sister do not have it, nor, as I once thought, did my parents Xavier and Nellie (they are shown the photograph below on their wedding day in 1941), or, as I once thought, did my grandparents on either side.

I know of no other biological relations - aunts, uncles, cousins, nieces or nephews - who are autistic, at least not noticeably so. I do believe that I would recognize it, now, in any of them if it were there.

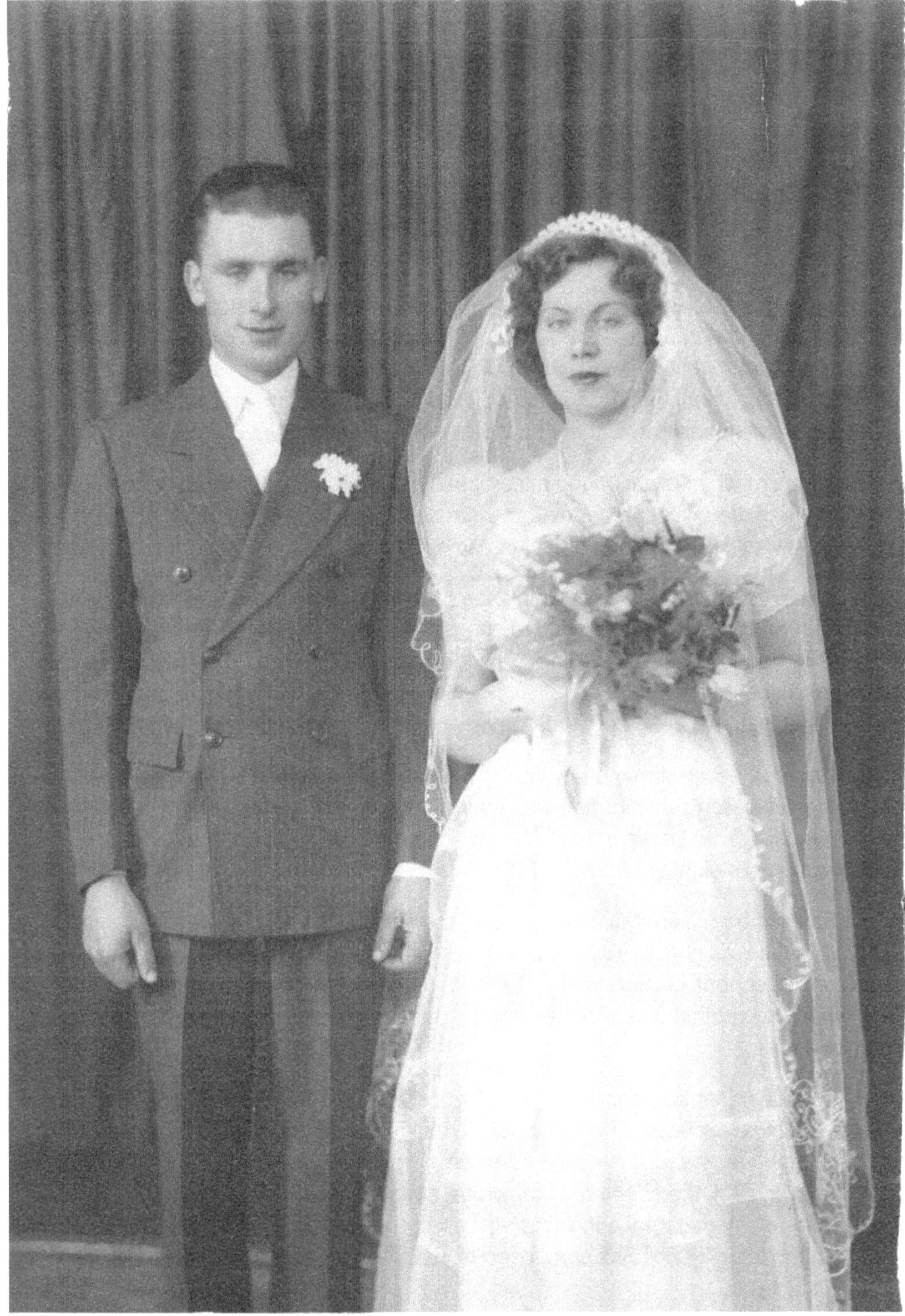

Recognizing The Signs

I have, however, since my own awareness happened, begun to suspect that *a particular line* of my direct ancestry was somewhere "on the spectrum." It may be that it is only after the light, a particular wavelength on the spectrum (i.e. as with visible colors) the awareness of one's own condition, has been switched on that one is able to see what has always been obvious. It's like seeing a color that has never been seen before.

My maternal grandfather had a sensitivity to loud and sudden sounds that almost everyone at the time regarded as just a quirk "when Grandpa was cranky." I now wonder if he was "cranky" because of how, and why, such sounds (e.g. a slamming door – which, as it happens, is the same one that can make me "cranky" too – even the same door in the same house that I now own) were affecting him.

Our judgment of why he was made miserable by sudden loud sounds may have been a mirror image of the actual reason – both were visible, but it was our view, and ironically then, my view still, of the cause that was backward

His daughter, my mother, as I now think back, while apparently not affected by loud, startling sounds (I think it reasonable to suggest that *everyone* is to some degree bothered by "loud racket" – especially if sudden and unexpected), did have some habits and peculiarities that I now recognize in myself. She was a kind and friendly person, but in a way that was markedly different from my much more sociable Dad. *Just like me*.

The photograph below is that of my Dutch-Belgian born mother as a teenager. My maternal grandparents immigrated with their two daughters and a son (my mother was the middle child, born between her older sister and her younger brother) when my mother was about eight years old.

My mother was born literally in the middle of the First World War (1914-1918) in time and place. She was born in 1916, half-way through the war, in Flanders where some of the major battles took place (the war poem *In Flanders Fields* was written about the place where my mother was born, referring to the time of war there in my mother's hometown area).

When I was doing family genealogy years ago, it was my mother's line that happened to become the most successful in my search. Thanks to a distant-related monk (a *sixth cousin*, or *sixth degree* as it is stated in Europe) in a monastery near my mother's home town (the town clerk there, where I first wrote, directed me to him), I have the identities of every one of my maternal ancestors all the way back to 1596. For over 400 years, for most of them, their "world" was composed of just a few adjacent villages in Flanders.

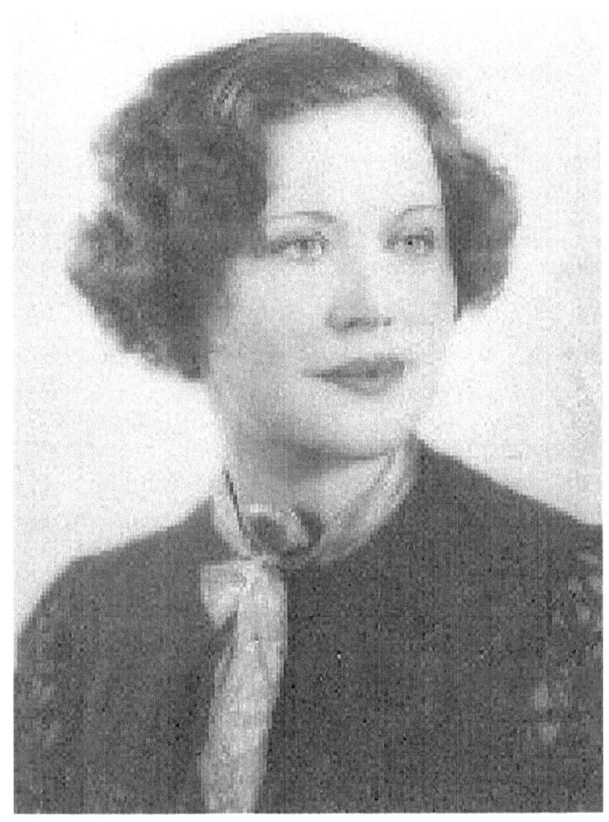

Were my grandfather and my mother autistic to some mild degree, or carriers of it through the centuries? I now think that the possibility is strongly there.

When my father died, many people came to his funeral. When my mother died 9 years later (I was present in the hospital when they died, both of them from cancer – with my mother when my father died, and alone with her when my mother died – I literally saw her last heartbeat in the pulse in her neck), very few people came to her visitation or the funeral.

It was, as I now realize, like a proverbial "elephant in the room" hint of *why* that solitary exit happened.

It is only now that I can *see* what I was looking at. I had time to think about that when I sat, alone, with my mother at the funeral home while waiting for her "friends" to show up for the visitation. It was as if the two of us were being alone together – she in death, me with no other living person in the room. Both of us autistic.

> ➢ **TIP** ~ I now wonder, if there were no God, if the oblivion of death would be the ultimate autism what awaits everyone. Logically and scientifically, I do however believe without doubt that there is indeed a God, a Supreme non-physical being who created all things. Without the design of set in place beforehand laws of physics, the "Big Bang" would have been the "Big Dud." But my over 20 years of daily writings on that can be found elsewhere.

If my mother and her father were autistic, that would suggest that autism, in some, may be heritable – or perhaps, the *vulnerability* to the condition is possibly inherited. Maybe both. I think more the former – the vulnerability, rather than a certainty of manifestation.

A Happy, Solitary Childhood

What about all of the other possibilities?

What about exposure to chemicals in the environment? Or vaccines?

I grew up on a farm in southern Ontario in the 1950s and 1960s in which chemical pesticides were just beginning to be used on a large scale in the agricultural industry throughout North America and the world (millions of people had the *same* exposure to those chemicals). It nevertheless did not seem to be having any serious obvious effect on anyone at the time.

The photo below of my mother, our dog "Duke" (he was a young stray that we adopted and kept until he died of old age at about age 16; I spent many, many hours exploring the farm and woods with my friend "Old Duke") and of a white cat that I don't now remember much about, was taken by me in the mid-1960s. As you can see, everyone looked happy and healthy on the old farm.

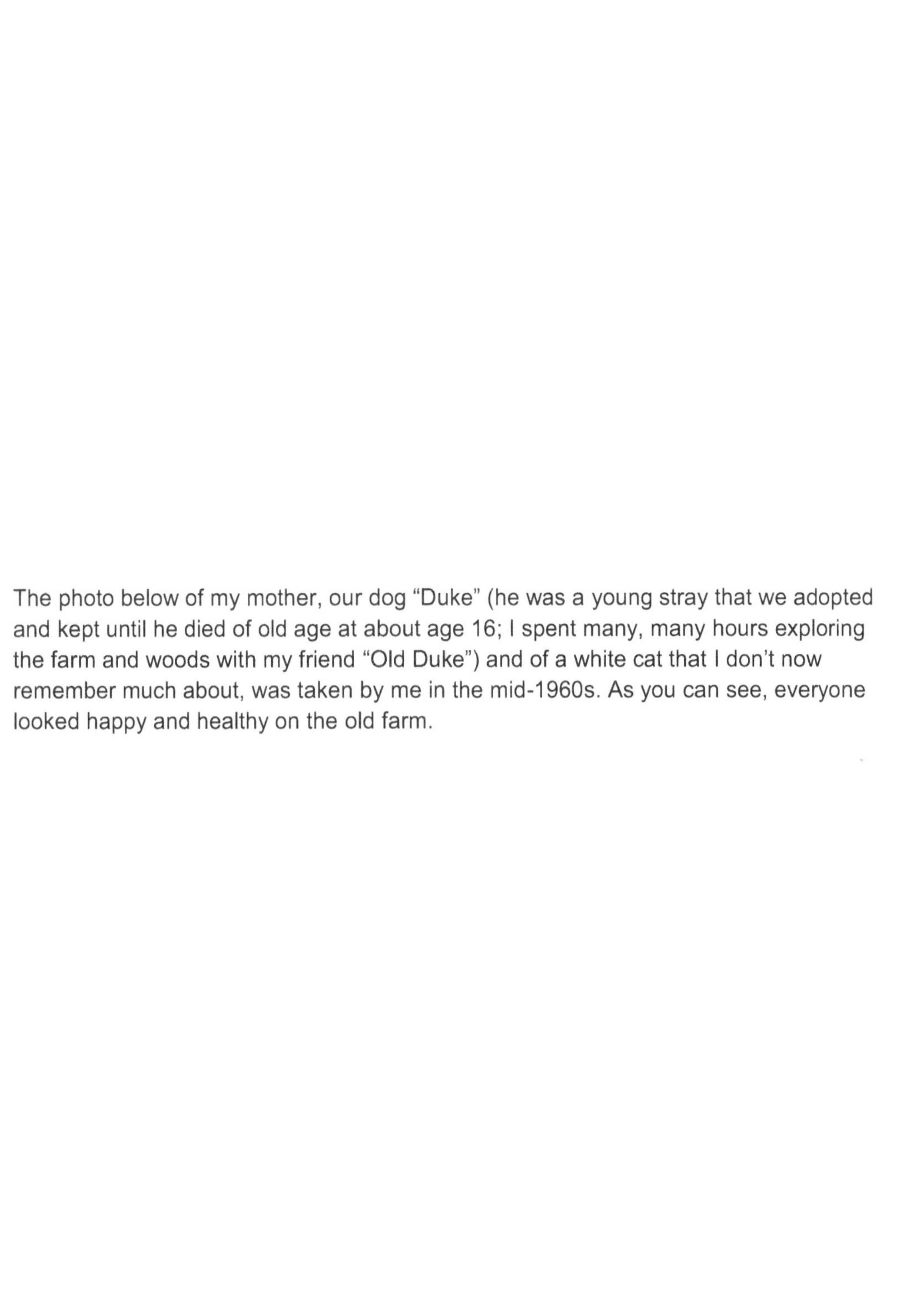

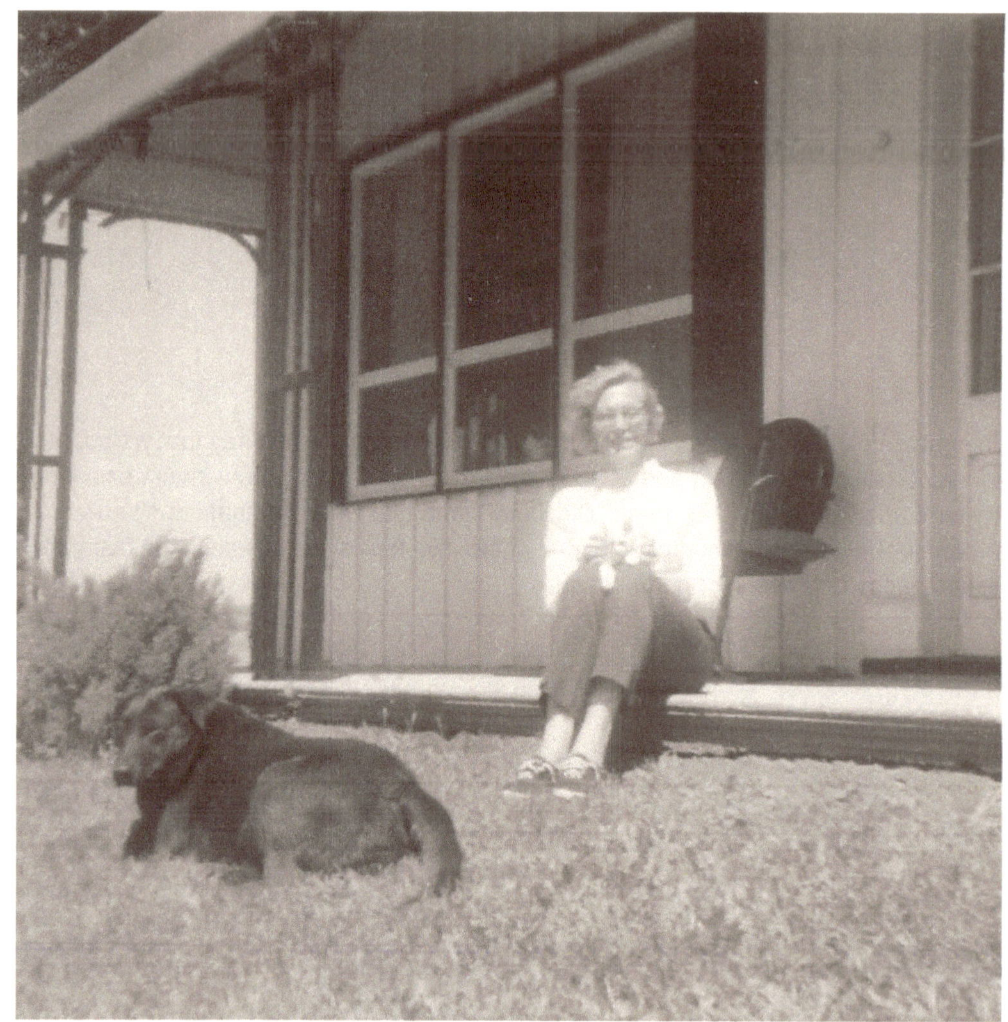

My mother would have had some exposure to those substances, as I also would have therefore before and after birth. My siblings, who were born in the early and mid-1940s had less exposure to those chemicals as infants, although the same exposure by the time that they were teenagers.

As an infant and growing child, I received the full range, at that time, of vaccines – *twice*. My mother told me that when the family moved from one farm to another, the family changed doctors (back when doctors routinely made house calls), which caused my first set of immunizations to not be completed – so the new doctor started them all over again.

It was sort of a family jest that I would never get any of the childhood diseases because of that repeated dosage. I didn't either, except for measles when I was about 12 years old – by which time, as I now realize, the autism was long present and active.

Otherwise, I had a very physically healthy childhood – no illnesses what so ever, except for the common cold that I nevertheless seemed to get less often than family and friends. I could hike for miles, play some sports as good as anyone does (baseball better than hockey because hockey requires two major skills to be done at the same time – more about that in the chapter about manual skills) and had very high grades in school – when I attended (more on those two points later).

I was happy, free and well cared for by loving parents. I thought throughout that time, and still do, that I had a blessed childhood. I grew into a strong young man of about 5' 11" and 170 pounds (my weight has remained at that level throughout my life, right to the present day).

On a general scale, while some might suspect the agricultural chemicals or repeated immunizations could have been a cause, that would not account for autism that existed through history long before those things existed. None of those things existed at all in the time of Bleuler and Asperger – while autism obviously *did*.

So, what does that prove?

No Single Cause, But Perhaps A Single Vulnerability?

If I were forced to make a nonprofessional's guess (albeit as an "expert" on autism because I live and breathe it) as to the cause of the condition, at least in my own case, I would say that it developed, or at least manifested itself, about age 2 (I will explain that in greater detail, along with a photograph that I believe provides proof, in a later chapter), due to my own inherited susceptibility for it. If it were more greatly a matter of simple inheritance, my brother and sister "should" have it too. But they don't.

A point that I now wonder about. My brother "takes after" our father (i.e. complexion, hair color, personality) while I am much more like my mother – not just in the sandy hair color, but in personality.

Is autism, or the vulnerability to it, not only heritable, but so in specific lines of siblings i.e. my mother may have been the only autistic one of 3 siblings, just as I am the only autistic one among the siblings (the 3 is, I think, just coincidental, but the line of transmission is not).

My sister looks very much like my mother, but personality wise, she, like my brother, is much more like our Dad. So I wonder, to what degree can unseen autism also determine personality?

But let us continue.

As I mentioned in an earlier chapter, I was well developed during pregnancy – born in September rather than the calculated due time in August. My fetal development was not rushed or stressed. My mother was a strong, healthy farm woman in her late 30s living in a peaceful place. My birth was without problems.

The only infant care difference that I know about is that while my siblings were breast fed, I was mostly bottle fed. The reason for that is that my mother soon went back to work on the farm during the busy autumn and winter season (my parents needed the money, and there was no "day care" back then), so I stayed with my paternal grandparents about 15 miles away.

I was bottle fed and cared for by that grandmother (my father's mother – my father was the oldest of six children) and two aunts (my father's two youngest sisters who were unmarried teenagers at that time) for about my first six months of life, rather than my mother who I only saw on weekends.

My mother told me how I would cry (and then my mother did too) when taken from my grandmother (who would cry) and then cry (and then my mother did too) when I was left by my mother with my grandmother at the end of the weekend.

Did that back and forth seeming "Who is my mother?" experience (I was never left alone however – there were always loving family members around) leave a psychological scar? I don't know. I doubt it. But I am certain that it had no effect what so ever on me being autistic. Autism isn't as simple as that, nor are its causes.

An "Extreme Male Brain"?

It seems from my observations that autism affects males substantially more than females – or perhaps more likely, autism manifests itself *differently* in males and females. While no longer "politically correct" to state that truth, there is still indeed a profound, primal biological and neurological difference between male and female brains and minds. Autism itself may be subject to those powerful differences.

The fetal development of male or female is itself an interesting study that may also explain the seeming differing rates, or manifestation characteristics, of autism between the sexes.

There is the old question, usually stated as a joke, "Why do males have nipples?"

But the answer is no joke. It's a reality.

Any fetus can develop into male or female when it receives its genetic instructions to continue. Males have nipples because they existed at the starting point, but they did not develop into females.

Almost everything is "standard equipment."

Other body parts could have developed into male or female in the same way. Ovaries could have descended and become testicles. The primal phallus could develop into either a penis or a clitoris. The folds of the labia may extend and then close and become a scrotum (the "seam" along the bottom of the scrotum, where the labia joined together during gestation, remains visible for life).

Some research suggests that autism reflects an "extreme male brain," because people with the condition often have, in extreme form, a greater number of supposed behavioral male traits e.g. mathematical proclivity, attention to detail in a way different than the female and a supposedly lower nurturing *nature* – what made males the hunters and defenders of a family, while the females were better mothers and caregivers.

I have wondered if blood type is a factor, or indicator, for autism. I do not know the blood types of either of my parents, or of either of my siblings, but I do know for certain, from tests done, that my blood type is the relatively-rare *A Negative*. Is it more common in autistic people – as a cause or an effect? I will leave that to be answered, or speculated upon, by the other kind of experts.

Does autism affect animals? Or is "autism" perhaps the *nature* of various animals. It seems to me that cats are generally "autistic" solitary creatures, while dogs are generally more social i.e. like "normal" humans.

I believe that nature provides many of the answers if we observe with an open and honest mind – and have the courage to ask the questions without fear or prejudice.

Chapter 3: A Gift Or A "Defect"?

Einstein and Newton

"Social impairment."

"Developmental disorder."

"Intellectual defect."

If I were inclined to be a little defensive (which I may be anyway – the reader may be the judge of that by now) about such labels, just why shouldn't I? Why shouldn't *anyone*? And particularly considering the kind of men who were the original focus (pun intended) of its study and "treatment"?

Are autistic people underdeveloped, or are normal people "over ripe." Perhaps I'm being a little critical (with no malice included) with that question, but let us consider how inaccurate such generalized labels not only can be, but surely are most of the time.

Were people such as Albert Einstein and Isaac Newton autistic? If you read their biographies or their personal writings, you could be led to the conclusion that they were somewhere "on the spectrum." I think that they were – Einstein *by his own admission* and Newton by his well-documented behavior.

Einstein and Newton could, by the way, be prime examples of another theory about the "cause" of autism – an excess of neurons in some parts of the brain. Such a concentration of intellectual power could therefore produce genius in some interest or activity – or a handicap because it could be, for some people, too much of what would be a good thing in lesser amounts.

Consider this quote from Albert Einstein's published essay, *The World As I See It* (originally published in *Forum and Century*, Volume. 84, in 1931). Stated in his own words, from *his own experience*, he is describing the "normal" life of many people with autism. It rings oh so true in my mind as well (even though I am certainly no "Einstein").

> "My passionate sense of social justice and social responsibility has always contrasted oddly with my pronounced lack of need for direct contact with other human beings and human communities. I am truly a 'lone traveler' and have never belonged to my country, my home, my friends, or even my immediate family, with my whole heart; in the face of all these ties, I have never lost a sense of distance and a need for solitude"

Note also, from the same essay, how Einstein describes how one's "own little world" can be a powerful, *beneficial* force for good.

> "It is the duty of every man of good will to strive steadfastly in his own little world to make this teaching of pure humanity a living force, so far as he can. If he makes an honest attempt in this direction without being crushed and trampled under foot by his contemporaries, he may consider himself and the community to which he belongs lucky."

Further, despite (or because of) Einstein's intellectual genius in theoretical science, he was a physically awkward, often poorly-communicating, professor in the classroom. His students sometimes found it a chore to listen to his in-person awkwardness because the communication of his genius was in what he wrote, not what he was able to speak effectively.

As someone with the "focus," I strongly suspect that Albert Einstein was autistic. His appreciation for what is "normal," and what is, but what is regarded as abnormal by a given majority in a place or time (remember the Ugly Ducking mention earlier?) may be seen in what is to me a very revealing part of what Einstein truly was in his mind and heart.

Newton Was More Extreme

Isaac Newton was, I believe, *severely* autistic. He experienced a more upscale version of the spectrum that crossed from genius to near disability – or in his case, were an at-times conflicting mixture of the two at the same time.

Newton, by coincidence or not, was born very premature – he weighed less than 3 pounds and was not expected to survive more than a few hours after birth. Those who believe in the not fully developed cause could perhaps cite Isaac Newton as an example. *But what then about everyone else?*

Newton, like Einstein, like all the others, was unique – not only in their choice of focus but in their degree of how it both empowered and, or, weakened them.

What Makes Genius?

But what accounted for their "genius" then?

It should perhaps first be kept in mind that "genius" simply means to be the first to do something or to be the originator. The words *genealogy* and *genesis* are on the same "spectrum" as genius. Perhaps another word would be more appropriate.

But were Einstein and Newton really greater in intelligence than the "average" person? Did their brains somehow have greater power? Or were they, by means of their obvious autism, capable of harnessing, *focusing*, their "normal" level of intelligence to greater power (like rays of the sun focused by a magnifying glass – more about that later too) through the concentration that is, I believe, the "cause" of autism behavior?

An example. If you were reading a textbook and watching an instructional video about another subject at the same time (I won't load the example by saying reading two textbooks at the same time, or watching two instructional videos at the same time), would you be doing either as well as you would have by doing them separately and alone? The answer is obvious, isn't it?

Now imagine if you could focus your thoughts on a particular task or problem in a way that most people could not, or perhaps, do not because they never learned to do so, or never do so because of *their* nature? Both Einstein and Newton went for days, forgoing food and sleep while *focusing* deeply on a scientific theory.

An ironic and tragic loss to humanity is that many with a more extreme condition of the "focus" may have been even greater in intelligence than Einstein or Newton, but humanity never benefited from it because they were never able to communicate their discoveries. Some may even have perished in Asperger's death clinic – Einstein *could* have.

Einstein's very life, if he had remained in Europe rather than fleeing when Adolf Hitler came to power, was endangered, *twice*, because of the "racial purity" fantasies of the Nazis. He could have been among the autistic children "euthanized" by Asperger, or he could have been killed in the Holocaust because he was a Jew.

How Many Autistic People Are Members of Mensa?

I am not a "genius." I believe that my intelligence is no greater than the average person. Years ago however I passed the Mensa Society entry test that would have enabled me to be a member of that group whose membership is limited to that of the top 2% of intelligence (based on various I.Q. tests).

I believe that I did that, not because I'm any smarter, but because I was able to focus on each question in such a way that the answer could be seen more clearly – there wasn't a lot of other "stuff" blocking the view of the desired answer.

I did not continue with it because it would have meant having to associate with people on a social basis. But ironically, I passed the constituted reason that the organization exists. That seems sort of funny, doesn't it?

There may be a paradox in that, but also, the reason that I mention it is that while autism may be the average person's way to "genius," there are obviously others who achieve it in another way.

Perhaps there should be a version of Mensa for people in the top 2% of *concentration* ability. If there were, it would likely be filled with autistic people – although they would not have the social gatherings in their society. Their "meeting" would only be attended by individuals, in many places around the world.

At the other end of the "spectrum" are those who, while they may be just as intelligent, or I think, usually more, are unable to effectively communicate with other people. They are what the definition of autism is commonly based upon.

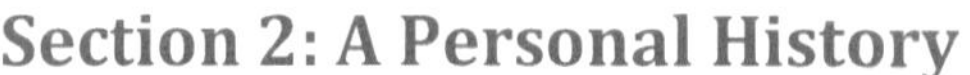# Section 2: A Personal History

Chapter 4: Birth Order: Cause Or Cover?

Family Life As The Only Child – With Two Siblings

I am the youngest of three children. My brother is about 14 years older, while my sister is about 12 years older. My parents were both age 38 when I was born.

I do not know if my parents' relatively advanced parental age had anything to do, as a matter of genetics or fetal development (if I was born with the condition) with my autism. Some may be of the opinion that it is, at least, a contributing factor – just as age can be a factor in a number of other conditions. It is a reasonable assumption, or perhaps, presumption.

I am however quite certain that their later time of life for me did contribute to my not being recognized as autistic much earlier. The same can be said for my happenstance elder siblings who were practically a generation ahead of me. I recall from my childhood occasionally feeling as though I had two sets of parents. Perhaps there were advantages and disadvantages to such a situation.

It seemed quite ordinary, even expected, for the youngest to play alone at home when, for example, his brother was age 20 when I was just starting kindergarten.

My parents were good people, loving and responsible to their children. I had a happy childhood. I loved reading and taking long totally-free hikes in the country (back in the "*good* old days" when it was safe to do so) and the surrounding woods where we lived on the farm. If I was happy, they were happy.

My within the family solitary existence (although never alone) seemed natural, as indeed it is for millions of "normal" (that word keeps happening, doesn't it?) siblings. But I now believe, in hindsight, that while just another common, coincidental experience, I think that it delayed awareness that there was something more involved.

The approximate decade and a half time gap between the births of my siblings and I could cause some to assume that my birth was an unintended surprise. But it was not. As a number of relatives (aunts, uncles and grandparents) attested, the birth of my cousin to my father's brother and his wife caused my father to want another child. He spoke among the family of it. I was born about 2 years after the birth of my cousin Ron who was the inspiration for the creation of me.

I was born "late" – calculated to have been a mid-August baby, but born overdue in the first week of September.

But still, those "only child" (i.e. my siblings were almost a generation older) circumstances may have made my autism seem "normal," almost expected.

Do you see why I believe that "normal" is a relative term that has at least of much to do with the observer as it does with the observed? I did not have to be autistic to live the childhood that I, and presumably millions of others have experienced. It is only when it became a matter of focus (no pun intended) on the child that it became a problem for others.

> **TIP** ~ Finding a way to be part of the focus is the beginning of communication with those with autism. *Join* in, don't break in.

That point of course would apply only to those who are "high function" autistic – a "normal" people's devised term generally defined as an autistic person with an I.Q. nearing that of "normal" people (apart from those with an I.Q. much higher than "normal" people e.g. Albert Einstein – but the definition, devised by "normal" people, tends to focus on those that "normal" people are "superior" to).

On the other hand, or at some other point along the spectrum (or in the "orbit"), those who experience it severely, as a handicap, would be more distant from the starting point. But the basis, the root, is the same for all. I am certain (if not also proof) of it.

But despite the solitary existence, I liked people. I liked being around people. I just happened to do it in a solitary way. I agree completely with Einstein's quote about that – he *knew* what one must *be there to know*.

Chapter 5: School Years

"Tom Sawyer" Threatened With Reform School

I began school in a typical of the time traditional one-room country schoolhouse that was located just a short distance, about a ten-minute walk, from the farm that my parents had purchased that year. There was one teacher for grades one to six, after which the children were bused to the nearby town for grades seven and eight and high school.

The children at the school were almost all farm kids from the surrounding area (back then, "homeschooling" had that additional meaning), so we were a homogenous group. Nevertheless, from that time, I often found myself more interested in spending the day exploring the nearby woods or creek – almost always alone. I developed a keen and intimate interest and knowledge of "nature" from that time.

I wonder if the "getting back to nature" expressed desire of many "normal" people is based on the same primal attraction that I felt as I actually did it. "Nature" is everywhere, the same nature. It is a greater freedom than any man-made "society," regardless of whatever "freedom" labels that are superficially attached to it, could ever be made to be.

"Playing hooky" began early, but no one did much about it. My grades stayed very high. I always passed the exams easily without having to go back and study my notes (much of which I didn't have anyway because I wasn't there – but I knew it anyway from experience or other reading – material usually far ahead of my grade year as I did my own "home schooling" too).

My report card, along with the many days absent, indicated a student who was doing well in traditional, institutionalized school. If I had been failing, the absence might have had to be dealt with much earlier.

I have since learned that all of the children were given I.Q. tests at that early age and that I scored very high – I had the second highest, or highest, score in the school. I know that because the teacher, Mrs. Johnson, in a moment of scolding my friend Eddy (as it happened, his sister married my brother a few years later) and I for throwing snowballs at the school wall, very close to the windows, that we had the highest I.Q. scores in the school, so "Why don't you two boys use your heads?"

> **TIP** ~ Autistic people like people and enjoy friends. It's just that they do so as though the friend is autistic too. Unfortunately, that almost always means that friendships don't last. With the missing social cues, the friend often interprets the relationship as a lost interest on the part of the autistic one, and so drifts away.

Due to declining enrollment, the old school was closed at the end of my grade four. All the children were then bussed to the nearby town to continue their schooling.

While my grades continued high at the new school, I missed the old country school – or rather, the country around it. I began skipping school even more than had been *natural* for me before i.e. it then also had a purpose.

It was then that I, as I now realize, had my first serious confrontation between my solitary autism nature and what the world of the majority demanded. "Playing hooky" then became known as the ominous legal term "truancy."

A Trip To The Woodshed

After a few unheeded warnings (by me, not them – perhaps the autism was preventing me from "hearing" what they were threatening, at least at first), my parents were given the official dire ultimatum, *a direct threat*, that if my truancy did not stop, I would be taken from them and be sent to a residential reform school, in effect a prison school, so that I would attend to my legally required education until I came of legal age.

It was a shock and embarrassment to my parents and an absolute terror to me. I was, in effect, at age eleven or so, being treated like a criminal for my free-spirit "Tom Sawyer" way of playing hooky – while maintaining grades higher than most of the children who never missed a day.

It was for that that I received the only "trip to the woodshed" (it was actually to the garage – we didn't have a woodshed) beating that I ever received from either of my parents. After being slapped and punched to the ground, I begged my Dad with a sobbing, drawn-out "Please" – to which my Dad repeated with a mocking tone and kicked me as I lay on the ground.

I could see in his eyes for days afterward that my Dad was deeply sorry and grieving for what he had done. I didn't blame him then, nor do I blame him now (he died over 25 years ago). I understand why he did it – and back then, it was common for misbehaving children to be beaten. Perhaps his sorrow was for the mocking of my begging him to stop. I don't know. It doesn't matter now anyway.

How much that violent incident, or how much my fear (I "got the message") of being taken away from my world were each a factor, from that time on I attended school without missing a single day – a perfect attendance record.

I focused on never missing a day, perhaps because I really had no choice, but also, or, because that school became my focus of interest. It really wasn't so bad after all. I attended even on the rare days when I had a cold or flu, and could have remained home without legal problems. Imagine having a child that insists on going to school. It was an "Every parent's dream" that my own parents enjoyed from that time on.

The result, however, was not what anyone intended. They forced me to be there physically, which I chose to do, but it ironically, as I can now see, took my autism to a higher *internal* level.

My teachers mostly regarded me as a quiet, diligent student – which I was in completing the work that they gave to the class (often in about half the time it took most of the others). But I was still playing hooky by going, then intellectually, anywhere that I wanted to go.

The books of the school library were my tickets and vehicles to anywhere and any time. I was farther away than I had ever been when I was merely physically absent. Ironically, all of that extra "escape" reading in the library also made me more all-round educated than would have otherwise been done if I had been content to be there in a "normal" way.

It continued on through high school and beyond through my entire life.

Getting The Strap

Back when it was permissible, even legal, to do so (the beating device could actually be purchased from school supply companies back then), I also got the "strap" twice during my school years. It seems violence was once regarded much higher than it does now in "proving" who is "right."

The first time was at the one-room school when I was about 10 years old. It was a very cold January day. While playing outside at lunch hour with my classmates I got frostbite in my earlobes. As anyone who has experienced frostbite, once a frosted or frozen part gets warm, the sensation isn't that of cold but of intense *heat* – it feels like a burn.

As it happened, the teacher was scolding us for throwing snowballs again. While she was doing that, the searing pain caused me to put my hands over my burning ears.

Perhaps some of the other children had some frostbite too, but to me that pain was *everything* that I could think or do about.

The teacher, when she saw me doing it, thought that I was trying to keep the sound of her upset, lecturing voice out of my hearing – so I was hauled up before the class and given the strap. I can still see that yellow-toothed crone (violence, it seems, gives people the worst possible views of the violator) as she jumped slightly into the air to put her full weight into the blows that she was inflicting on the child in her care.

She was inflicting *freaked-out anger*, not justice.

I went home that day with burning ears *and* burning hands. Nevertheless, in the eyes of the other children, I was a "hero" for weeks afterward They did not realize what really happened either.

Over the next week, the frostbitten ears swelled and the skin peeled as they were healing (the incident left no scars), making it obvious to some as to why I had been holding my ears that day, but the teacher apparently did not see it, or chose not to and admit her violent error in inflicting suffering upon suffering, pain upon pain.

The second incident happened at the new elementary school when I was in grade 8. The no-offense-intended blunt manner of autistic speaking or the tone of what is said (i.e. "It's not what you said, but how you said it") was misunderstood by the principal of the school as serious disrespect, so I was summarily taken into his office (which was next door to the library) and given the strap.

I can still vividly see the sadistic look on that man's face and eyes. Strangely, and perhaps appropriately so, it was very much the same countenance as the earlier incident with the female teacher in the old country school years before. For that few minutes, they had the same *spirit* of wanton violence.

While it is true that they did not know of my autism (I didn't then either!), there remains the valid question of whether *anyone* should have been treated in such a manner.

But it wasn't over. Upon leaving the principal's office after the beating, I put my hands into my pockets because of the throbbing pain in them – which the principal erroneously regarded as more disrespect (he viewed it as though I was nonchalantly acting as nothing happened), so I was literally dragged back into his office and given the same number of whacks again.

No hands in the pockets upon leaving that time – my throbbing raw hands were too busy wiping away the tears of pain – so I presume that he finally got the response that he wanted.

While the autistic tendency to remain silent, at least at times, when an explanation could perhaps have diffused, for example, those brutal situations, both of them may have been the seeds of my from childhood on belief that (paraphrasing the well-known saying) "Might *does not* make right" (again, Einstein's quote is right-on accurate).

Truth and what is truly right are not, in reality, based on the "law of the jungle" where the powerful naturally rule over the weaker that they seek as their subjects. In that regard, those painful and unjust incidents were character-building experiences – *good ones*, at least for me.

I may be autistic, but I am not a thug or a bully – even though I suppose that I have always been physically strong enough to be violent if I had chosen to take the dark road. I might have those lessons from the two teachers to thank for that peaceful nature. After all, ironically in their cases, aren't teachers supposed to *teach*?

Chapter 6: Relationships

The Age Of "Doing Your Own Thing"

I lived my teenage years in the late 1960s and early 1970s – the so-called "hippy" era. I was typical in appearance and behavior as that of millions of others. But always, something more and more noticeably *different*.

I was also at times, extremely reckless – driving much too fast and skydiving lessons. The only fear that I got from either of those activities is when I now think back at how foolish and flagrantly reckless they were. They terrorize me *now* when I think about it. Life is so precious.

But with young adulthood also came *sovereign* autism. Even at that relatively young age, I really did not care about anyone's approval for my personal choices of belief or behavior. It wasn't a matter of rebelling against something because I was never by choice part of most of it.

I recall going to a particular rock concert. A number of times, those in the audience, thousands of young people, stood and clapped or danced to the music. I was enjoying the concert too, but I remained either seated or stood without the arm flailing or hand clapping. I enjoyed being there just as much, but all in my own way.

The signs were becoming less subtle, perhaps some even *deliberate* – even though it would be many years before I could really see them myself. I didn't yet know *why*.

Like millions of others, I experimented with marijuana (which became legal to use and possess in Canada in October 2018) and some of the other drugs on a very few occasions. I was never a "drug user" as so many others. I never really much enjoyed the effects of those substances. They interfered with my clear view. I had the saying, "Dope is like a dirty window."

My favorite drugs were however beer and cigarettes. I no longer consume any kind of alcohol (more about that in the later chapter about social inclusion), and I quit smoking in my mid-twenties after smoking for about a decade. I never actually enjoyed smoking, nor do I think that most people do either. Most of my years as a smoker were actually years of trying to quit that very addictive weed.

The satisfaction that many say they experience from smoking may be entirely a matter of satisfying the demands of the addiction within themselves – smoking is a *relief*, not a pleasure. It is the addiction within, like a parasite that is actually doing the smoking, in a way, using the person to do it. That may be true for all addictions, of substance or behavior.

I knew many young women during that time. None of the relationships lasted, but then the "free love" spirit of the time made that seem normal too. Another coincidental and convenient cover.

The only exception to that was a girl that I dated and was engaged to, for about four years. We loved each other, but she ended the relationship because of my supposed jealousy – that began when I found her drinking at a bar with another guy when she thought that I was at work (I was at work, but on the way home saw her car parked near the bar).

I wasn't as much angry with her as I was disappointed to see her, not with another person, but *as* another person. It wasn't a matter of something having changed. It was a matter of coming to see something, someone, for what they actually were. It was over well before it actually ended.

Jealousy Or Loyalty?

A word about "jealousy." To an autistic person, that means *loyalty*, not possessiveness or control. Autistic people could perhaps be some of the greatest proponents of personal freedom (some historians have suggested that Thomas Jefferson was autistic). But they are also, at the same time, some of the greatest proponents of loyalty and fidelity.

Consider some examples of autistic "jealousy."

As mentioned, I witnessed the deaths of both my parents, of cancer, in the hospital.

My father was the first to die. My mother and I were with him when he died. Their two "normal" children were *not* present. Just the autistic one *chose* to be there.

When my mother died about 9 years later, I alone was with her. Again, like my father, their two "normal" children were *not* present. Just the autistic one *chose* to be there *again*. Without him, my mother would have died completely alone (as I likely will someday too).

My sister was not there, either time, because, through no fault of her own, she was too far away to get there in time. She would have been otherwise. Autistic people don't have a monopoly on loyalty.

When our father died however, my brother wasn't there because he was "busy" and "couldn't get there in time" - from a 30-minute drive away.

My brother was also not present at the death of our mother despite then living even closer (about a 10-minute drive, in the same city) than he was to the hospital when our father died. He knew that she was dying because I called and told him. But he stayed away. *He did not even go to our mother's funeral even though he was still just as close.*

Many people in the family were shocked by his absence. Some have asked me why he did it. My answer is that I simply do not know. I never asked him, because I have never seen him since – by his choice. I have tried repeatedly, by email, telephone, letter and by a third person, but always no reply.

Finally, I accepted his will and have never made any further effort to contact him. I would however still very much welcome hearing from him.

I will not judge anyone for their choices, or their supposed reasons and justifications for making them, but I record it here merely to make clear that the loyalty of autistic people is almost always *unconditional* loyalty, right to the end, even when things are no longer convenient or pretty. Autistic captains go down with the ship. Autistic people don't just leave people to die – especially their own parents.

If such dedication is a "defect," so be it. But what does that say about what "normal" has become? Perhaps the world would be a better place if such "developmental impairment" *loyalty* were the norm.

More about that in the chapter about marriage.

Chapter 7: The Discovery

How I Discovered That I Am Autistic

A few years ago, I met a lady from Connecticut through my website. She was a rare exception to my inability to reply to communications. As it turned out, she had a major effect on my life's awareness.

She was divorced with two sons. One of them served in the U.S. Military as a paratrooper in the 82nd Airborne in both Afghanistan and Iraq – he enlisted not long after, and because of, the 911 terrorist attacks in New York and Washington. He bought his mother a beautiful marble chess set while he was in Afghanistan (she was in charge of the chess club at the school where she worked), which I now have (I will explain why in a moment).

She was an intelligent, highly educated woman who worked as a librarian at Middle Schools in Connecticut, including one only a few miles from the Sandy Hook school at Newtown where the horrendous mass shooting happened in 2012. The perpetrator of that evil event was diagnosed with Asperger's Syndrome - a condition that is related to autism.

I have never been able to understand what drove that young man to do such a thing because most people "on the spectrum" are definitely *not* violent. But I mention him only because it was by means of that woman in Connecticut that I discovered that I am autistic – *peacefully* so. It was a shock to both of us.

As I look back at that relationship, I am amazed at the ironies of it. The odds against how that happened seem very high.

Over time, she became more and more upset with my "stubbornness" (as she called it) until one day, based on the autistic behavior that she was confronted within me, when neither of us realized that I was autistic, she angrily accused me of being a *narcissist*.

A narcissist?

I wasn't familiar with what narcissism involves, so with an open mind, I read as much as I could about it. I knew immediately that I did not fit what I was reading – most of the traits of narcissism are actually directly opposed to the benign traits of autism. I told her that. But she refused to believe it.

So, to satisfy her insistence, I got tested. I was right. I am *not* a narcissist. But I scored very high on the autistic scale in every test that I took. Over and over and over again.

That was how and when I discovered my autism.

It was a *shock* ("What, *me* not "normal"?"), but also a relief. It explained so many things throughout my entire life.

The awakening also could have given me an excuse for some of the bad things, but I refuse to do that. I believe in accountability, regardless of mitigating factors.

On my parents' gravestone, below their names, is engraved "Rest In Peace." Whenever I'm there to visit, I now include "*from Wayne*" in my mind as I read that line. I caused them a great amount of stress and grief for which I am now, too late to do anything about it, very sorry.

But other kinds of peace came. I no longer struggled to improve or correct what was *me*. I would have to become someone else to do that. I do not like fakes either.

By that time however, it was too late to continue the relationship. She married another man a couple of years later and we each moved on to new relationships.

But more irony. Our being together for the rest of our lives would not have happened anyway.

At about the same time that she was married to another man, she discovered that she had Stage 4 kidney cancer. Despite the most advanced methods of surgery and cancer immunology treatments at the Yale Cancer Center, she died in 2018.

She was buried in a small family plot overlooking the Connecticut River.

Knowing of my love for playing chess, "unlike anyone else I've known" (she said), she willed me her marble chess set that her son had brought from war-torn Afghanistan on a U.S. Military transport aircraft. I have it here to this day.

Section 3: Understanding The Experience

Chapter 8: The Focus

Is The "Focus" Good Or Bad?

Those who become the best at something do so because they dedicate their lives to it. Athletes are an example. Runners *run*. Golfers *golf*. Every day. They *focus* all of their time and energy on what they do in order to become the best at what they do.

Focus, of itself, is not a bad thing. It is the key to success in many things. That may be regarded as the good side of "focus."

> ➤ **TIP** ~ To an autistic person, focus does not mean self-centeredness. Perhaps one of the greatest ironies of autism is that autistic people tend not to be *selfish*. It's not part of the experience.

Consider these amazing quotes about focus by those who became successful *because of it*.

- "Concentrate all your thoughts upon the work at hand. The sun's rays do not burn until brought to a focus."
  Alexander Graham Bell (1847-1922), Scottish-born Canadian and U.S. scientist, inventor of the telephone.

- "My success, part of it certainly, is that I have focused in on a few things."
  Bill Gates (1955 -   ), a founder of Microsoft Corporation

- "You can't depend on your eyes when your imagination is out of focus."
  Mark Twain, pen name of Samuel Langhorne Clemens (1835-1910), writer and humorist.

- "It is during our darkest moments that we must focus to see the light."
  Aristotle (384-322 BC), Greek philosopher and scientist.

- "Planets move in ellipses with the Sun at one focus."
  Johannes Kepler (1571-1630), German astronomer and mathematician.

What happens if a focus becomes such an extreme that it negatively affects other things or other people? When does the classic "absent-minded professor" become a danger to himself or to others if he cannot see or hear what, or who, is going on around him?

Isaac Newton was a prime example of such a genius who was so focused on his work that he went without proper eating, sleeping and personal grooming for days at a time. There is no doubt that Newton made great contributions to science, but would such behavior today be tolerated by the "normal" people who might regard Newton as being a danger to himself?

Therein is both the gift ("high function") and the disability of focus. They are also, I believe, examples of the underlying impetus of autism.

Many are of the opinion that autism is increasing in our day. Estimates of 1 person in 100, or even 1 in 40 have been suggested in popular news media. I believe however that what they all ignore is that *everyone* is autistic, one way or another.

I am not attempting to normalize autism, because in this world *solitary* autism is a definite minority "problem." There is though the reality of what I have come to call "singular autism" and "group autism." If you appreciate this, you are opening the door to understanding that autistic people are not different, but rather are manifesting their autism in a singular way that leaves everyone else out.

Group Autism

How can there be such a thing as "group autism," a single focus in a group of people?

> If you have ever been in the military, you've experienced it.

> If you work at a company (consider the multiple meanings of that word) with other people, you have experienced it.

> If you have been a teenager, you have experienced it.

In each of those examples, participants are expected to be *of one mind*, members (plural) of the single-purpose team. Those who don't or won't are regarded as abnormal and rejected. They don't have to be singularly autistic to have it happen.

I include teenagers in that because, regardless of the generation, in them it can be seen most strongly. Each "individual" is expected to dress similarly, speak the same and have the same tastes in virtually everything. How many actually do, but put his or her true self aside in order to be accepted is a question that can be answered by almost everyone who has grown up to sovereign adulthood. They almost *all* do, except perhaps for their "leader" who decides for everyone else.

An Attention Deficit?

The classic "attention deficit" of autism is also a paradox in that those with such a strong ability to focus their attention are very often unable, not unwilling, to focus, to pay attention, to other people or things.

The problem, however, isn't just a matter of refusing to pay attention to others, but rather already having a *filled* capacity, which is often larger than that of the one they are seemingly ignoring.

> ➢ **TIP** ~ If you want an autistic person to pay more attention to you, find a way to make yourself part of the focus of attention. But a happy warning! Once you do, you could find yourself looking for ways to reduce it.

The Source Of Genius

As mentioned earlier, the ability to focus everything on one thing provides a return of greater achievement. Newton's famous falling apple would have been worthless if he had not at the same moment been focusing on a theory about gravity.

The actual apple incident was recorded by Newton biographer William Stukeley in 1752 in his *Memoirs of Sir Isaac Newton's Life*. An excerpt:

> "After dinner, the weather being warm, we went into the garden and drank thea [i.e. tea], under the shade of some apple trees… He told me, he was just in the same situation, as when formerly, the notion of gravitation came into his mind. It was occasion'd by the fall of an apple, as he sat in contemplative mood. Why should that apple always descend perpendicularly to the ground, thought he to himself"

What if Newton had been focusing on something else when he saw the apple fall? What if he had been thinking about lunch rather than physics? Would the famous incident then have been about apple pie?

Are Autistic People Liberal or Conservative?

Most autistic people tend to be apolitical. But what if they weren't? Would they more likely be liberals or conservatives?

"Conservative" means to conserve what already is. "Liberal" means to liberate from what already is.

By literal definition, all revolutionaries are "liberals" who violently refuse to conserve the established order. Ironically, or somewhat paradoxically, they immediately become "conservatives" of their newly established order.

Most autistic people are, by nature, paradoxically, "conservative" (they don't want or need a change) *and* "liberal" (they are not part of the established order to begin with).

Chapter 9: Why So Much Repetition?

Striving For Perfection

Repetition or lining things up in a particular (usually perfectly straight) way is a classic symptom of autism. I used "is" in the previous sentence because they are in fact the product of a single purpose.

The photograph below shows the farmhouse (built about 1810 by pioneers from England, successively modernized over the over 200 years of its existence) that has at the present time been my home for many years.

The previous owner was my widowed mother (more about that house later), and both of my parents before that. My mother sold the farmland around it and had the house lot of just less than 2 acres legally severed so that she could keep the house while selling the land.

After I became the owner, I planted the hedge around it. The cedar and spruce trees were about 6 inches tall when I planted them. As seen in the photograph, they have since grown tremendously.

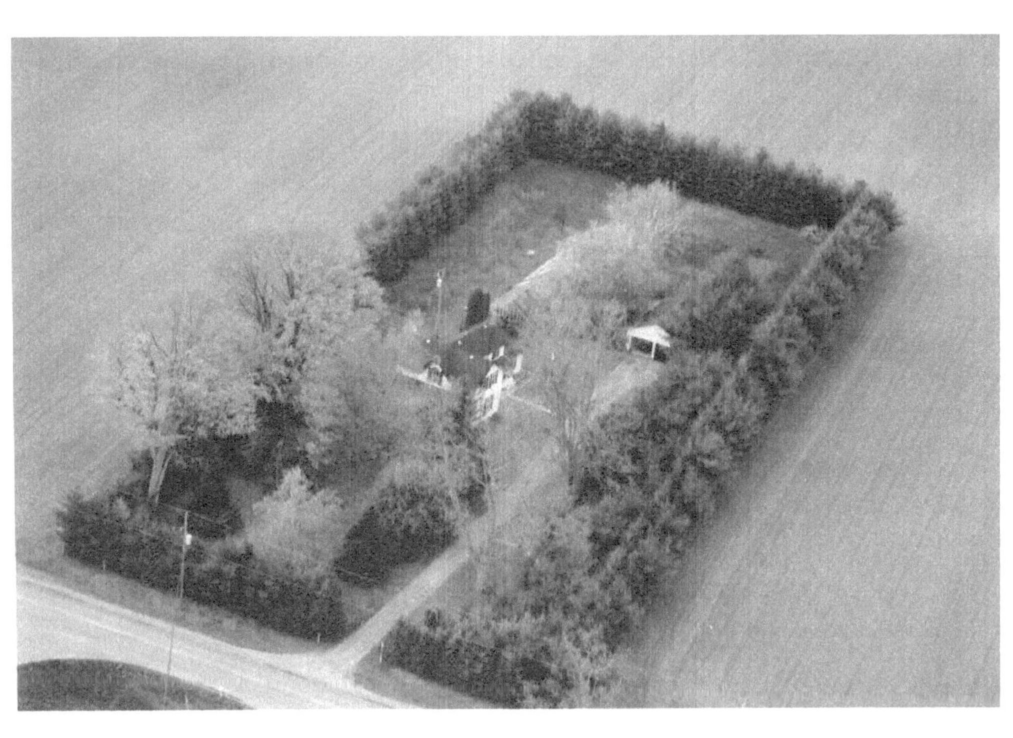

I have, since I discovered my autism, come to sometimes jokingly refer to that barrier (that all sorts of songbirds now also call their home) as my "autistic hedge" - for a number of reasons.

An autistic person planted it. As can be seen in the top tips of the hedge trees, it was planted perfectly straight, like an autistic child lining up his blocks or toys. But moreover, without yet realizing it at the time, the autism made its own statement by my planting it between my *self* and the world.

Lining things up identically is itself a repetition But repetition is not tho point of doing it. It is a *striving for perfection* that being firmly focused on something demands. The repetition happens when a perceived flaw, or even an interruption, is discovered or encountered.

> ➢ **TIP** ~ Repetition by autistic people is due primarily to perceived imperfection. The flaw is that it causes all that is "perfect" up to then to be discarded. Rather than the last bar of a piano piece that alone needs more work, the whole is discarded and restarted to learn.

Before I realized that I was doing it, that is, *why* I was doing it, I read many books only part way and started over again "to get it right this time." The problem, of course, is that perfection does not exist in life such as it is. At best, we can work to perfect ourselves, or something that we do, without ever arriving at perfection itself.

So too when I was learning to play the piano. The theory was easy. The playing skill was hard work that demands daily practice (I still play today) to remain sharp (no pun intended).

But my problem came in learning any particular piece. Any mistake would provoke a re-start of the entire piece.

Mistakes often naturally happen at the end, like a runner slowing or stumbling at the end of a long race. I was only able to overcome it by perfecting a piece bar by bar. Then, like blocks placed in a straight line, I was (usually) able to play the whole piece "perfectly."

The same re-starts happened with my learning of other languages, primarily Dutch (i.e. for my maternal ancestry) and German (for my paternal ancestry), but also with French and Hebrew that I am to this day working on.

That, I believe, is the way that most autistic people can achieve what merely appears to others as repetition. It is not a perfect perfection, but the method works very well for me – not just in now finishing books or new piano pieces, but almost anything that I want to focus on for a while.

As with so many other ironies, autistic children are usually very strict about putting their toys neatly away – while "normal" children typically leave their toys scattered everywhere, to be tripped over on the stairs, or to be run over in the driveway. In that regard, most parents might very much appreciate a little "autism" in all children!

> ➢ **TIP** ~ You can lessen the repetition by recognizing and supporting what is right. Encourage the perfect parts and you might find that the repeats will get shorter because the restart will begin at a later point – rather than realigning all of the blocks (repetition) only those farther along will be repeated.

There are no simple or easy answers, but there is always a way to make things better.

Chapter 10: Sound and Fury – Sensory Overload

When A Good Thing Becomes Too Much Of A Good Thing

Autistic people can be oversensitive, or under sensitive, to a *very* wide variety of things because their senses of hearing, touch, smell, sight or taste typically take in too much information at once, or not enough information fast enough. In that way, every autistic person is unique i.e. their body settings are "autistic" too.

It's the "focus" that makes an autistic person more sensitive, because they're focusing on it, or less sensitive because they're focused on something else (the classic "absent-minded professor").

That situation can be either a special talent or a crippling condition. Having an "eagle eye" talent would be very useful for someone doing lookout work, or having acute hearing would be beneficial to an ornithologist who is seeking the presence of a particular kind of bird in the dense forest.

> ➢ **TIP** ~ Almost anything can be too much or too little to an autistic person. The key is to recognize particular sensitivities and to avoid them as much as possible. Like the doctor who told his patient "Then don't do that!" in response to their complaint "Doctor, it hurts when I do this…"

Loud or sudden noise, bright or flashing light, clothing of a particular texture feeling, a temperature that is too warm or cool are all common sources of distress because the senses (vision, hearing, touch, smell and taste) take in too much or too little information.

> ➢ **TIP** ~ One extreme is just as distressful as the other. Replacing distressful loud sounds with silence can sometimes simply transfer the distress from one extreme to another. As with so many other things, healthy *moderation* is often the answer (think of the *Goldilocks and The Three Bears* children's story in which the porridge was either too hot, too cold or "just right."

Pain, or lack thereof, is another. I never had any problem with normal pain levels. The frostbitten ears and strap incident long ago showed me that they were working very well.

Many experience different, specific overloads. For me, it's loud and sudden sounds or "racket" in general. Loud alone isn't a big problem for me. But the very same sound can actually be *painful* if it happens either suddenly or maliciously.

I remember an incident as a teenager in which the door (as mentioned earlier, the same one that caused my grandfather such distress – but I never made the connection until years later) below my upstairs bedroom was slammed so hard that it hurt. I ran downstairs and screamed at them, pleaded with them, to please not do that. It was like an explosion, perhaps not in the door, but in my head.

My Dad didn't appreciate being told what to do in his house, plus my way of saying it, so he responded by waiting until I returned upstairs and then slamming that door, over and over again – deliberately because of what I had said, or rather, how I said it.

I don't hold it against him. He didn't know about the autism, or how painful that sound was to me. And I probably did say it in a seemingly disrespectful way. And it was his house.

I now own that house – and that big, heavy door. Some may wonder why I didn't remove it when I got the legal right to do so. But it wasn't the door's fault. It is actually a nice, antique door built many years ago, perhaps even with the house when it was originally built in the first decade of the 1800s. The problem was my autism, not the door. But if you're wondering, no one slams that door now in *my* house.

> ➢ **TIP** ~ The problem with autistic overload, of any sort, may not be as much a matter of experiencing something, but being *forced* to, whether by suddenness or a deliberate act. For example, you might like eating popcorn, but would you like it at all if someone forced you to eat it? Would it not then be a stressful experience for you?

I now commonly wear industrial foam earplugs used by, for example, people using power tools, along with the sound muffs used by people who work at airports or at gun ranges. The two give me the auditory peace that I need, when I need it. I don't wear them all the time, but, as it happens, I'm wearing them now as I write this.

When I was younger, loud music was not a problem if I were playing it on "the stereo," or listening to it live (i.e. in a bar when I used to drink beer). The problem only happened when it was sudden or startling – or a deliberate act of cruelty by someone who through no fault of his own didn't know any better.

Chapter 11: Communication

Why Can't Most Autistic People Communicate Effectively?

As covered earlier, I continue to have some difficulty in replying to written communication in a timely manner. But I rarely have a problem replying by telephone.

I could go on a car journey and ride for hours without saying anything to the person that I was with – and yet still be very much enjoying the *company*. The other person of course, if "normal," would likely find the experience uncomfortable.

> **TIP** ~ Autistic people aren't ignoring your presence or your words. They are merely experiencing them as they are. Carl Sagan, in his *Cosmos* series, described how if someone from a fourth-dimensional universe visited people on three dimensional Earth, the humans might, for example, be able to hear the fourth dimension being, but not be able to see it even though it is there. In some ways, "normal" people are also alien in how they are perceived by the autistic. This would be most pronounced in those with "severe" autism, but the principle exists for nearly all.

I could talk with the lady in Connecticut on the telephone for hours at a time. Rarely was there a problem when we communicated in that way. When we met in person however, it was often an awkward experience.

In fact, our first meeting in person turned out to be no meeting at all. She *surprised* me by just showing up at my door – even though we had specifically agreed to have our first meeting at some later day. I refused to open the door.

She then called me on the telephone, by which we spoke with our cell phones, even though we were just a few feet apart with a door separating us. That seems so ridiculous, almost comedic – although neither of us was laughing. Without intending to be philosophical, the "door" (another door) of course was the autism.

It was from that embarrassing incident that she sought some sort of answer as to why I did that. That humiliating blockage (most people would have ended it right there) never stopped bothering her. Or me.

Her eventual answer, after experiencing more strange-to-her responses, was narcissism, which led to the discovery of autism.

> **TIP** ~ Being pressured to meet the will of others, or to be surprised by someone who wants something, is a major roadblock to communication for the autistic. It doesn't open doors; it closes and locks them.

I emphasize though that the problem there was the surprise, not the meeting itself - being forced to communicate in a way that, apart from our agreement not to do so then, turned out to be one of my primary symptoms of autism.

Albert Einstein (and I reiterate, I'm no "Einstein") had it too. He is world famous for his writings, but those in his in-person classes, or public appearances, very often had a very difficult time "connecting" with him. It seems very possible that if Einstein wasn't who he was, he would have been fired, or at least kept out of classrooms and speaking halls.

Another common communication problem is interrupting. That is something that I have done all of my life – and only now do it much less because I am aware of it, and why I have habitually done it.

In my own case, it was/is due to an *overwhelming* urge to share a thought that comes to mind as I hear others speak. To me, waiting would make it less relevant or meaningful. It isn't about trying to be rude or dominant in conversation.

 As always, there is a reason.

> **TIP** ~ Autistic people often interrupt others while they are talking. It isn't intended as a matter of rudeness or aggressiveness. It is a matter of either not recognizing when the other person has passed the turn to speak, or being unable to suppress a response that "can't wait."

My learning to control things such as interrupting is not intended to suggest that there is a "cure" for autism. That kind of "surgery" would require the removal of the person's existence. It does, however, suggest that improvements can be made, particularly when one focuses on doing them.

A "problem" can be turned against itself to produce something better, perhaps like forest firefighters deliberately starting a controlled fire that will make a nothing-to-burn barrier to the oncoming greater fire.

The tone of voice, or even a monotone voice, is another problem area for the autistic. The "It's not what you say, but how you say it" factor. Intonation can be perceived as hostile or offensive when it is not intended to be so.

I assume that particular problem exists in all languages and all accents within each of them. As such, it provides an interesting conundrum.

Countenance, not smiling, is misinterpreted in the same way as intonation. I recall many times how I cause a smile to go away from the face of someone simply because I gave them a "Blank" look or stare (sorry, I couldn't resist the pun) in return. It wasn't meant how It seemed to look.

Fake smiles, however, make it worse. So are egotistical "show off" smiles in which people display their teeth or dental work as though they're doing a toothpaste or dentist commercial. There was a time when smiling like that was considered rude. In some places in the world, it still is.

People have even been bitten by dogs who "naturally" regarded the toothy smile as an aggressive snarl.

Eye contact too can be mistakenly viewed as suspicious or threatening. That doesn't just mean no eye contact, but also too much eye contact – what appears to be an intense stare.

> **TIP** ~ For those *severely* affected by their inability to communicate, a good general approach to conversation, or at least being "heard," is to say their name in a warm way, let that "sink in," then gently specify what you want, let that "sink in" too, then when comfortable, do it.

Autism is a very complex condition in which extremes are common. But again, that doesn't make it impossible to understand or live with.

> **TIP** ~ If vocabulary limited for someone with severe autism, use a few keywords – focus yourself on quality, not the quantity of communication. Build upon that when and if you can.

Chapter 12: Manual Skills

Multitasking Is Not An Autistic Strength

It would seem obvious that someone who naturally focuses on one thing cannot naturally do two or more things at once – not very well, or not at all.

It's like the old "Can't walk and chew gum at the same time" saying, while nevertheless being able to walk *or* chew gum better than most "normal" people.

> ➢ **TIP** ~ Focusing on what an autistic person does well is a key to helping them (if they need any help   there are many very successful autistic people In the world, as we will get to) be self-sufficient members of any society. Don't waste time and emotion by trying to fit the proverbial square peg into a round hole. It's foolish to try and certain to fail – unless the square peg is physically maimed (in the case of a living human being, psychologically maimed) to make it "fit" in.

Motor Coordination

Along with the focus factor, some may wonder if autistic people have poor motor coordination i.e. they can't make their hands do, or do fast enough, what their brain is telling them to do.

I don't think that the motor coordination theory is a problem for me. I can type on a computer keyboard as well as anyone. I can play the piano as well as most amateur home players can do.

I do recall that I was better at some sports than others. Perhaps that's simply the way it is for all people, but moreover, I was better at baseball than hockey. The reason for that *may be* because hockey is actually two sports in one – stick handling and skating.

However much the "focus" was involved, I also recall that I could hit a pitched baseball better than most because I knew where it was going as much from the pitcher's release as its trajectory. The same with catching a hit or thrown ball – I looked more at its launch than its flight.

As we will cover in a later chapter on that subject, autistic people do very well at some kinds of manual work, while not being able to do other kinds very well, or at all. For example, they might work well at assembling something to a very high degree of precision or quality because of the concentration that is required, but be unable to do it if it were on a moving assembly line or with some sort of a time deadline – or with someone "supervising" them in an overbearing sort of way.

More on that in a moment.

Chapter 13: Social Cues and Signals

Forrest Gump

Perhaps the primary "problem" that the "normal" world has with functional autistic people is that they are socially clumsy. Their timing is bad. They miss cues. And sometimes, despite it all, they do well – which sometimes makes "normal" people even more upset with them.

It was only after I was given to realize the autism in myself that I could see the autism in others. As discussed, my mother and grandfather were real people, but I also then began to recognize that some fictional characters that I was familiar with were *portraying* autism. That is to say, the creators and writers of those characters were using autism to create an entertaining spectacle from which lessons could also be learned.

A familiar to many people example of that was *Forrest Gump* from the 1994 U.S. movie starring Tom Hanks, which was based on a book written by Winston Groom in 1986.

While most regard the character as being intellectually challenged, I believe that it was moreover autism that he had (keeping in mind that he was a fictional character, but what he portrayed was real-life autism – Tom Hanks did a magnificent job in that).

Gump was an honest, social klutz who was not actually "stupid." He was *different* in the way that he connected to the world. The success that he seemed to repeatedly stumble into was more than just chance. His greatest advantage in that regard was not knowing any better than to stay away from places of *opportunity* that "normal" people feared to go. He often won by default in that way. Maybe there's a lesson for everyone in that.

Gump's being able to play ping pong so well was because of his ability to focus on the ball – again brilliantly portrayed by Tom Hanks with those intense eyes. He knew where the ball was going long before it got there. Some of us can relate to that very well.

The hockey player Wayne Gretzky (as it happened, he was born in Brantford, Ontario in the same hospital that I was, about a year or so later) is said to have a "sense" of knowing where the puck will be, and then going there while everyone else is headed in the wrong direction. I don't think that Wayne Gretzky is autistic, but his "focus" in that way is, I think, a good example of how autistic traits are found, sometimes with much success, in "normal" people.

Mr. Spock

"Mr. Spock" from the original *Star Trek* series also displayed many autistic characteristics (that is to say, the writers used that fictional character to display autism), but with a revealing difference.

On Mr. Spock's home planet, the also-fictional planet Vulcan, everyone was like him. He was "normal" at home, but "abnormal" (although professionally respected) to Earthlings. On Vulcan, the normal people of Earth would be the abnormal ones. As I mentioned earlier, stepping across a line, however close or distant, can make you seem like something opposite from what you were one step back.

Alcohol

I actually find it humorous now that there is a "cure" for autism, at least for some people – alcohol. Alcohol made me "normal" – and foolish. And sick ("hangovers" seemed more intense that visibly experienced by the others).

While alcohol is commonly known to release inhibitions in everyone, it also, for some, makes them "normal" sociable (i.e. "social able") people, appearing to a large degree without autism.

I find that to be a paradox – that the autistic have to become unreal in order to be normal. I am referring of course to any pharmaceuticals that may be prescribed by medical professionals to "cure" people of their "Einstein" condition. Consider that carefully, and decide for yourself if that would be a good thing.

Honesty

The *portrayed* characters Forrest Gump and Mr. Spock were literally honest and truthful (Does it seem strange that both of them needed to be portrayed with that characteristic for them to be them?). They meant no offense, but they often caused it.

> ➤ **TIP** ~ Autistic people tend to speak honestly and literally. Unlike "normal" people they have much less motive to lie to or insult anyone. It's not part of their world. In the world as a whole, however, such as it is, truth, however well-meaning, is not often appreciated.

I remember years ago autistically (as I now know it was) blurting out to my brother in law, "You're getting fat," which immediately erased the smile from his face and caused him to reply, in a low, displeased tone, "That was not very nice."

But I didn't mean it to be offensive. He *was* getting fat, but I meant it as an expression of how well his business was prospering and how healthy he looked. I meant it as a compliment, but he received it as an insult.

So the question, would autism be such a problem for others if literal-speaking honesty was a common characteristic "normal" people?

Chapter 14: "That One's A Loner" – *Now*

Solitary Bliss And Blessing

I remember a comment that my Dad made to a friend who was visiting him. I was in the room when he said it, but I remember that I was being described more as an object than a living human being. He said, "That one's a loner."

He was right though. By then, I was exactly that. A "loner."

It apparently was not always like that, however. The picture below of my Dad and me was taken in January 1956 when I was about 17 months old (my mother kept that picture in her wallet for over 50 years – I inherited it when she died at age 86).

That photograph is one of the major reasons that I believe that my autism did not begin to happen before birth. Nor did it happen as a child who later received vaccinations or some other suspected cause that has become popular. It began, or *began to become active*, I suspect, not long after that picture was taken.

Why do I believe that?

Notice the happy smile, the direct eye contact, the warm appreciation of being held – all traits of a "normal" child, not an autistic one.

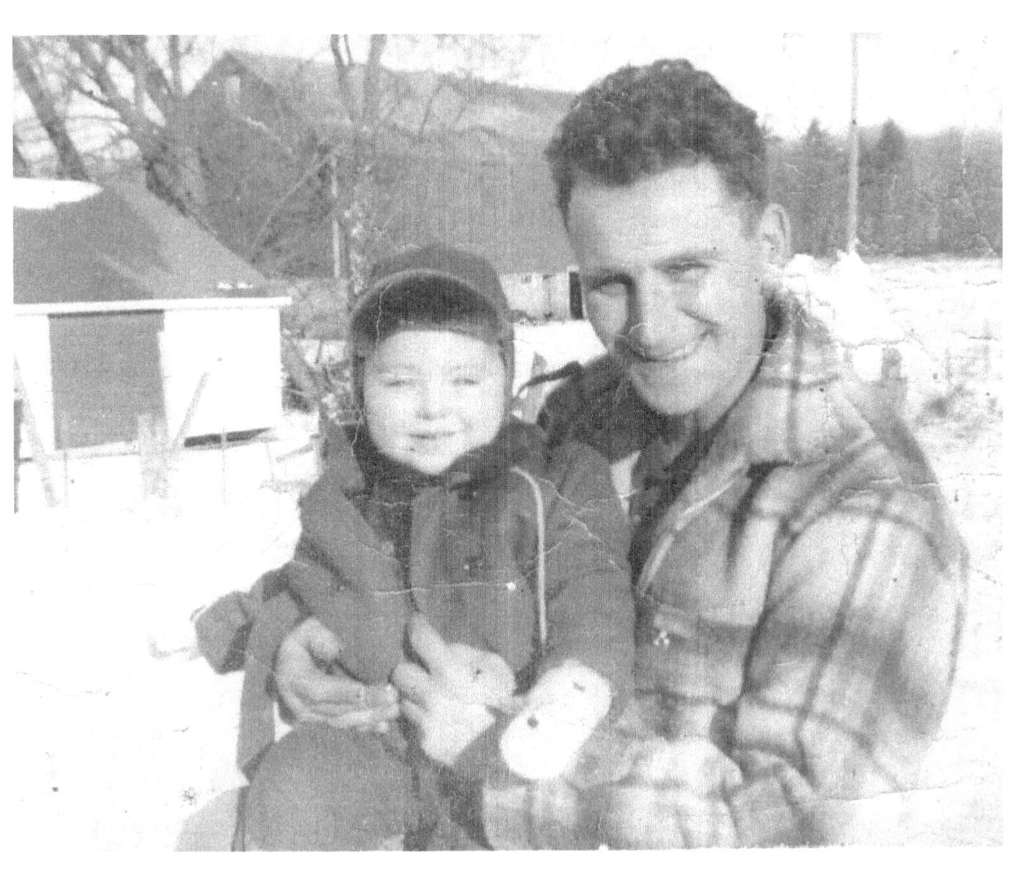

Although I have since never had many problems with being touched or hugged, it's also something that I now have no need for. When that picture was taken, I think that I did.

> **TIP** ~ Reluctance or refusal to be touched is a common trait of autism. It may not be as much a refusal as it is a difference in how being touched feels – physically or psychologically. But every individual is exactly that.

Solitary Confinement Wouldn't Be A Punishment

I recall another fictional character (I used to watch popular TV shows, but hardly watch TV at all now) that I regard as portraying autistic characteristics. Kwai Chang Caine on the early 1970s *Kung Fu* series was a solitary-minded man who found no distress in being alone in the wilderness.

I recall one particular episode in which he was arrested and thrown in jail for defending himself. He deliberately broke the rules so that he would be thrown into solitary confinement. The scene ended with the jailer snarling at how he would suffer in his solitary cell, but as the jailer then left, Caine was shown smiling (something he was rarely shown to do in that show) with satisfaction from being put there – as he intended to have happen. Only an autistic person would look at it that way.

What About Those Who Suffer From *Not* Being Autistic?

This book is not a defense or promotion of autism. Along with the few who may benefit from it, there are many more who suffer, without realizing it, from it.

But I believe that there are autistic qualities, that *everyone* has, that would be beneficial to them if they could somehow turn them on when needed. By that I mean helping people with loneliness in society.

Could autism be a cure for loneliness?

How many people today, such as the abandoned and left alone much of the time elderly (of which there are many in the world), would benefit from a mild case of not being distressed from being alone? *That* attribute of autism? Rather than losing their interest in living, giving up, they could have years of happy, even productive, life if they could be naturally set free of their "normal" distress from loneliness.

Section 4: Financial Matters

Chapter 15: The Autistic Person In Business

Why So Few Autistic Lawyers, Politicians And Used Car Salesmen?

Autistic people tend to speak and hear *literally*. As such, dishonesty and outright lying is generally alien to the autistic nature. It's "goes against the grain" as the saying goes.

What does that mean in the "real" world? Could someone who tends to be honest, too honest, be a success in a world that often isn't honest at all?

A good salesperson knows that to be successful one must tell people what they want to hear, to "puff" the product or service and never speak of any problems or flaws.

Autistic people would not do well in that regard. That's a generalization I know, but the nature of the condition is opposed to those methods.

Another factor is deciding what to sell. The worldly answer, of course, is whatever people want. "The customer is always right" in that regard.

But an autistic person, logically and honestly usually sees a genuine and beneficial need for something else. The view may be entirely correct, but selling it may be a total failure.

Although autistic people are capable of great financial success in the world such as it is, running a business is usually not something that works.

Successful People

Many famous and very successful real people of the past and present have been suspected of being autistic to some degree. Consider just a few from that category:

> Charles Lutwidge Dodgson (pen name Lewis Carroll) – Author (*Alice's Adventures in Wonderland*)

> Charles Darwin – Scientist and author (*On the Origin of Species*)

> Emily Dickinson – Poet

> Bobby Fischer – Chess Grandmaster

> Thomas Jefferson – U.S. Politician, President

Michelangelo – Artist, scientist

Wolfgang Amadeus Mozart – Composer of classical music

None of them were employees, directly, of the work that made them famous and successful. But none of them were successful business people either.

Some believe that Bill Gates, a founder of Microsoft Corporation and now one of the richest men in the world, is autistic. The "flat" tone of his voice, his declared "focus" work style and his rocking back and forth slightly when he's thinking deeply about something are all common autistic characteristics. While Mr. Gates is most definitely a success in business, it was his non-business work that propelled him to that height.

Coincidentally or not, Steve Jobs of Apple had the same characteristics – and the same success.

Autistic people generally make very good computer programmers, while most people find such work tedious or boring.

Financial success from "genius" should not be mistaken for being a "genius" at running a business.

An Autistic *and* An Artistic Genius

As someone who loves playing (average player, good, but not great) the piano, I have long been a fan of Glenn Gould (1932-1982). In my opinion, he was severely autistic, so much so that his weakness almost, at times, canceled out his strength.

Gould had an annoying (to many people who otherwise liked his work) habit of humming loudly as he played – not in practice, but in actual recordings or concerts. He was apparently able to get away with it because he was a genius (I believe most definitely an autistic *and* an artistic genius) who made great music. But I think that it hurt his commercial success. Perhaps, he didn't even know that "he" was doing it as he played because he was so much "at one" with the sound. Maybe that's why he did it.

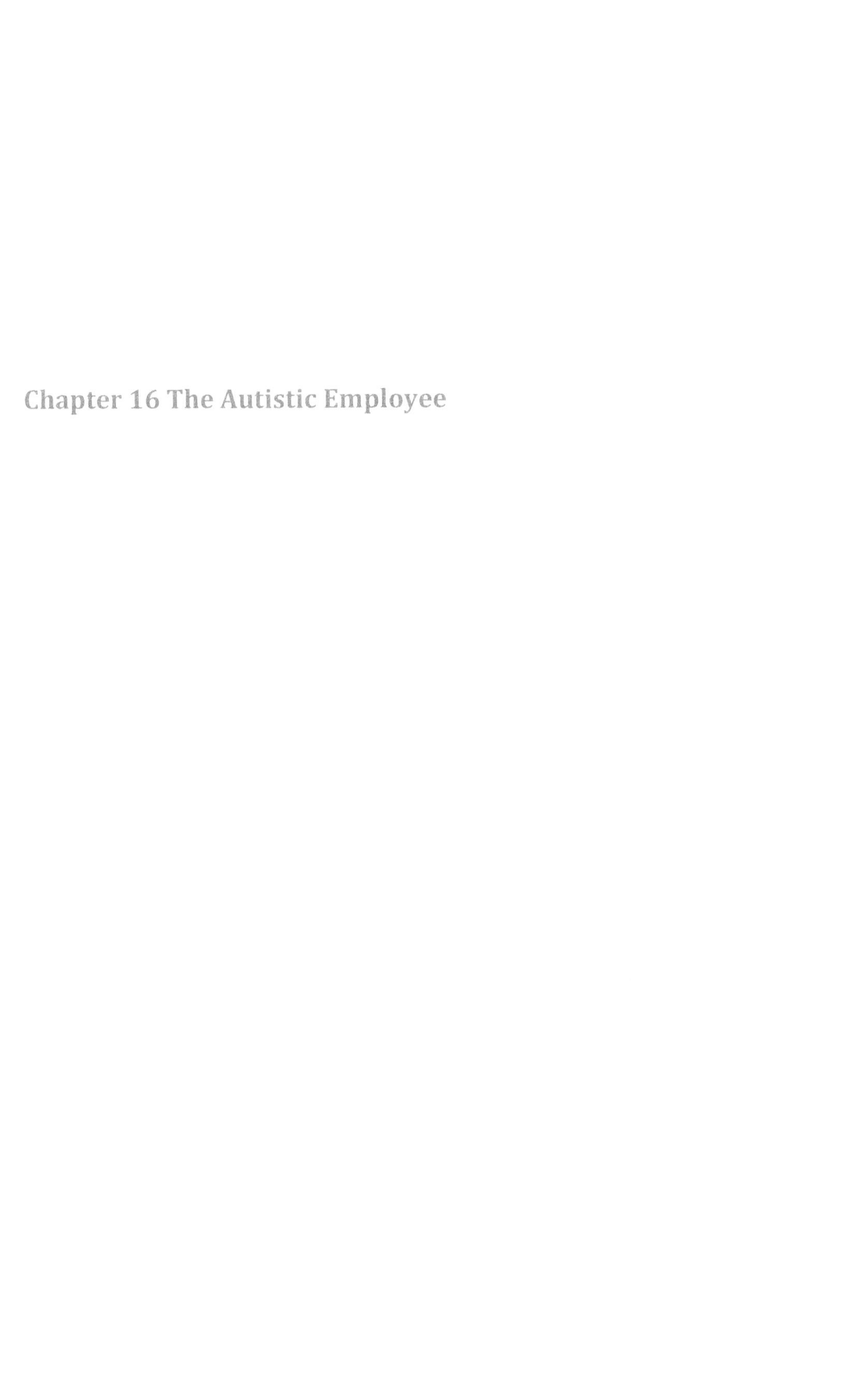

Chapter 16 The Autistic Employee

The Employee Worth Their Weight In Gold

On other hand (see the previous chapter), an autistic employee can be a valuable asset to any company *if* the right fit is found.

If you own a business, imagine having an employee who very rarely misses a day of work, won't steal from you or lie to you, does high-quality work – all while being a dedicated and loyal worker because of their focus.

That can happen if the focus is the focus of the work.

Software companies have had very good results with autistic workers (again, think Bill Gates), as have other companies in general.

In 2017, Ford Motor Company, Microsoft Corporation (surprise, surprise), SAP (another large software company), the bank J.P. Morgan Chase and others formed the *Autism at Work Employer Roundtable* to encourage the hiring of autistic people.

Why? Because they know the high business value of a functional autistic employee.

Many autistic people are needlessly unemployed, particularly since many are highly educated and want to work. The interview is usually the biggest barrier, but when the awareness of the autism is there, it quickly becomes obvious that the candidate has much more to offer than just a superficial, personable interview skill.

> ➢ **TIP** ~ Autistic people generally "Don't know how to act." They present themselves openly and without any facade. That is generally not appreciated at job interviews.

After hiring it's usually just a matter of accommodating any special, but usually very simple and inexpensive, needs for an employee (e.g. shielded from loud or startling noises, or music, or other employees who would behave aggressively toward them because of the typical autistic personality of directness or perceived lack of a sense of humor i.e. they don't laugh at foolish behavior or vulgar jokes) who would return that effort with a valuable human asset for the company.

They may not be a "team player" in the interpersonal skills sense, but they can be a valuable and appreciated member of the team.

Section 5: Life With An Autistic Person

Chapter 17: Parents and Siblings

The Dynamics Of Family Life

The place and circumstances of an autistic child in a family group may depend mostly on the structure of the family itself. Circumstances often determine other circumstances.

Is it a single parent family?

Is it a second marriage family in which the autistic one is a child of only one of the parents?

Is the autistic one the only child? Or the oldest? Or a middle child? Or the youngest?

Is there (as in my own family) a substantial age difference between the autistic and the "normal" children, whether much younger or much older?

With a little consideration, it becomes plain that they may have a very different life, or those in the family may have a very different experience, depending on how the family is structured.

The Reaction Of The "Normal" Children

Regardless of the overall circumstances, it seems reasonable to say that the autistic one will be the "focus" of the family due to the special needs, or problems ("normal" children may be reluctant to invite their friend over due to the presence and behavior of their autistic sibling), or benefits, presented by the autistic one.

"Normal" children may feel neglected or ignored due to the care demands of their autistic brother or sister. It typically causes them to "grow up" sooner than their years.

My Brother-Son

In my own situation, my sister was my sister and my babysitter. She was about 12 when I was born, 16 when I was 4 and 20 when I was 8.

I recall at least once when I was taken shopping with my sister when she was complimented on "what a nice son you have." She laughed, and I think that she genuinely enjoyed the misunderstanding. Perhaps it was her way of feeling "grown up" as most teenagers seem in a hurry to do.

As I stated earlier, I have not seen my brother since the day before our mother died in 2002. I haven't seen my sister either, after the day of our mother's funeral.

I wonder now if their refusal to see me was the "payback" for all of the years that I may have seemed to them as the family focus – or the trouble that I caused them. Neither of them knew of the autism, just as I didn't. But they surely knew and experienced that there was something more to it.

A Threat To Challenge The Will

Before my mother died, she announced to me one day that I alone was the Executor of her Will. She told me at that time that the reason that the other two children were not Executors was simply a matter of practicality. My brother had been spending six months of the year far away in Costa Rica (and didn't come around much when he was around much – the signals that he wasn't going to attend her funeral were there years before) and my sister lived about 400 miles away in another Province. I was here, so I was it.

That's really all there was to it. It wasn't a matter of taking control of an ongoing process in which decisions had to be made.

The Will itself was simple and brief. My mother's money (not a great amount of money) was divided equally among the three children, and her home was bequeathed to me alone. The reason for that was an earlier agreement/promise that my mother offered to me.

Due to severe arthritis, my mother was not able to tend to the large house and lot herself by the time she reached 80, so instead of "going to a home," she happily stayed at home (while emphatically saying that she did not want to "go to a home" while "my home is here") while I tended to the care and maintenance of it.

If that agreement hadn't been made, the house itself would not have even been included in the Will because the money from its sale would have been spent on expensive nursing home care for my mother.

When the Will was just about to be carried out, I was told by my mother's lawyer that my sister had hired a law firm, known for its aggressive tactics, to challenge the Will. Her totally-false accusation was that I had written the Will myself and was then trying to pass it off as genuine.

My mother's lawyer knew that wasn't true. The Will was written in his office and witnessed by his staff. I wasn't ever there and had no say in the contents of the Will what so ever – her lawyer knew that. The Will was then stored in that lawyer's office safe where it remains to this day. I have never even seen that original, only the official copy that I was given to me after my mother's death.

After a few stressful months, my sister withdrew her false accusations and threats to challenge the Will. Her own lawyer told her what she was accusing me of was false and impossible.

One way for one, and another way for the other, perhaps based on the same resentment of their troublesome little brother over the years, I have seen neither of my siblings since our mother's passing. That is not my choice.

I would very much love to hear from them – if only to invite them to read the explanations in this book. They still might not want anything to do with me, but at least they would then know the *why* of so many things.

Chapter 18: Husbands and Wives

Getting Beyond The "Courtship" Barrier

Autistic people often remain single simply because they tend to not be very good at "courting." The typical autistic personality isn't usually regarded as "attractive."

Some autistic people do marry, however. Perhaps the "normal" one is attracted to some other quality (maybe the classic "strong silent type" has its autistic version – if it didn't originate that way) that enables them to get beyond the possible barrier.

Then, the happiness, or the unhappiness, begins.

Feeling Ignored Or Enjoying Your Own Space

The success or failure may depend thereafter on what the "normal" spouse wants or needs.

If the marriage was embarked upon with the plan to "cure" the autistic one and "live happily ever after," it's not likely to happen. The normal one will be in a frequent or constant state of feeling ignored – even though the autistic one *isn't* ignoring them.

On the other hand, if the normal one is someone who wants to be married, but also needs their own independence and "my own space," they are likely to have a very happy marriage in that regard.

"Normal" people who have been married for a substantial length of time (when they become less saturated with the "love is blind" hormones) typically come to appreciate that situation too. It's *natural* for everyone.

> ➢ **TIP** ~ In my opinion, a key factor in a happy marriage to an autistic person is a common interest, talent or profession – if not at the start, then developed. That shouldn't be difficult or unreasonable since those who marry, regardless of who they are, should already have that working for them. It's called *compatibility*!

Autistic people are not alien to love or marriage. They just experience it differently.

Chapter 19: Children

More Autistic Children Than Autistic Parents?

Some might wonder if there are more autistic children than autistic parents. In a way, it's a reasonable question. In another way, it's illogical.

Perhaps we would be able to answer the question with certainty if there were some sort of "autistic census" done in which an actual count of autistic parents and children were known, but that seems unlikely to ever happen – I think, for the good. Data like that is, I think, a little too convenient to the people like Bleuler and Asperger of today.

Nevertheless, theoretically, more of one than the other could provide a strong clue as to the origin, or origins, of the condition.

If, for example, autism is a matter of simple genetic inheritance, how would that be represented in the parents versus children count?

Of if the cause were some outside factor that did not involve genetics, how would *that* be represented in the parents versus children count?

Or (also very interesting) if so many autistic people remain single, why are there so seemingly so many autistic children today? Where are they all coming from?

The Long View

There is little doubt that autism has existed through the ages – certainly much longer than just the past century when vaccines and pesticides were invented.

Autism knows no borders of time or place. To me, that strongly suggests a genetic, not necessarily "cause," but an inheritance of vulnerability.

If that view is correct, the ratio of autistic parents and children should be about even e.g. in my own family, I had two parents and two siblings, but of that family of five, only two people were affected by autism – *one* parent and *one* child.

Chapter 20: Friends

A Loyal, Intelligent Friend

Generally speaking (I might be his exception), my brother is very much like our Dad in his acceptance of people's differences. Whenever someone acted differently, he had a saying "It's just the way he is."

Autistic people can be very good to have as friends. The basis of a happy friendship is very much like that for a happy marriage. If you like company, while appreciating your own quiet space too, an autistic person is a good place to find it.

Despite, or because of, my autism, I have had many friends throughout my life. All of the friendships eventually ended because almost always they moved on with their lives while I remained in my own.

I like people. I enjoy company. But I can't go beyond what I am and how I am.

Like my brother says, "It's just the way he is."

Conclusion

A "Cure"?

Will a "cure" ever be found for autism?

Should a cure ever be found for autism?

The answer to that may depend more on the cause than the result.

If it is a matter of simple inheritance that makes it a natural state of existence for the functionally autistic, then the answer would seem to be *no*.

If it were a matter of a toxic effect of some substance that makes someone into who they would not have otherwise been, then the answer would seem to be *yes* – even though it's impossible to turn back the clock and have the "cured" person begin their life all over again.

And of course, if some means was found to lessen the too-extreme experience of those for whom autism is a handicap, then the answer would be a definite *yes*.

For me, the answer is *no*. Although I have lived most of my life without knowing that I am autistic, and despite the shock of when it was discovered, I would not want to be "cured" of being *me*.

I have always been the way I am. I'm very happy *here*.

Thank You For Reading

I hope that this book is helpful to you, whether you are an autistic person, a family member or a friend, or a medical professional with the willingness to better and much deeper understand what you are treating.

Autism is not alien to humanity. It is how many members of humanity were made to be *human*.